RUSHING WOMAN'S SYNDROME

The impact of a never ending to-do list on your health

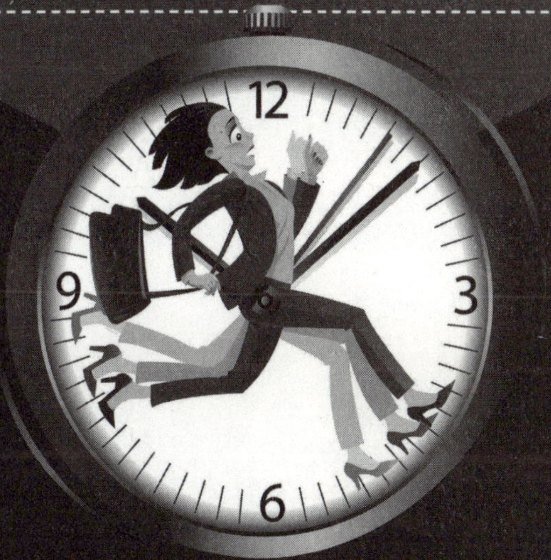

DR LIBBY WEAVER

Author of the best-selling book *Accidentally Overweight*

Disclaimer

The contents of this book are for information only and are intended to assist readers in identifying symptoms and conditions they may be experiencing. This book is not intended to be a substitute for obtaining proper medical advice and must not be relied upon in this way. Always consult a qualified doctor or health practitioner. The author and publisher do not accept responsibility for illness arising out of the failure to seek medical advice from a doctor. In the event that you use any of the information in this book for yourself or your family or friends, the author and the publisher assume no responsibility for your actions.

Published by Little Green Frog Publishing Ltd
www.littlegreenfrogpublishing.com

ISBN: 978-0-473-20403-7

For Christopher with so much love

&

For Kate with so much gratitude

RUSH

intransitive verb

1 : to move forward, progress, or act with haste or eagerness or without preparation

2 : to advance a football by running plays

transitive verb

1 : to push or impel on or forward with speed, impetuosity, or violence

2 : to perform in a short time or at high speed

3 : to urge to an unnatural or extreme speed <don't *rush* me>

4 : to run toward or against in attack : charge

5a : to lavish attention on : court **b :** to try to secure a pledge of membership (as in a fraternity) from

noun

1a : a violent forward motion **b :** ATTACK, ONSET **c :** a surging of emotion

2a : a burst of activity, productivity, or speed **b :** a sudden insistent demand

3 : a thronging of people usually to a new place in search of wealth <a gold *rush*>

4a : the immediate pleasurable feeling produced by a drug (as heroin or amphetamine) —called also *flash* **b :** a sudden feeling of intense pleasure or euphoria : THRILL

Origin of RUSH

Middle English *russhen,* from Anglo-French *reuser, ruser, russher* to drive back, repulse, from Latin *recusare* to oppose — more at recusant

First Known Use: 14th century

Related to RUSH

Synonyms: accelerate, bundle, fast-track, hasten, quicken, hurry, speed (up), whisk

Antonyms: brake, decelerate, retard, slow (down)

Merriam-Webster's Collegiate Dictionary

Table of Contents

Our mission is to educate and inspire people, improving their health and happiness, and, through that process, create a ripple effect that transforms the world.

Dr Libby and her team

Registered Reader

Congratulations on purchasing
Rushing Woman's Syndrome!

The science and understanding of the impact that nutrition and lifestyle choices have on our bodies is constantly changing as colleagues in the research world continue to make breakthroughs.

By purchasing this book you qualify for our Registered Reader program. Our aim with this Registered Reader program is to ensure that we are able to keep you abreast of the latest developments in health and well-being, as well as provide you with a touch point to continue to motivate you to achieve the goals you desire for your health and body.

Please become a registered reader
by visiting:
www.rushingwomanssyndrome.com

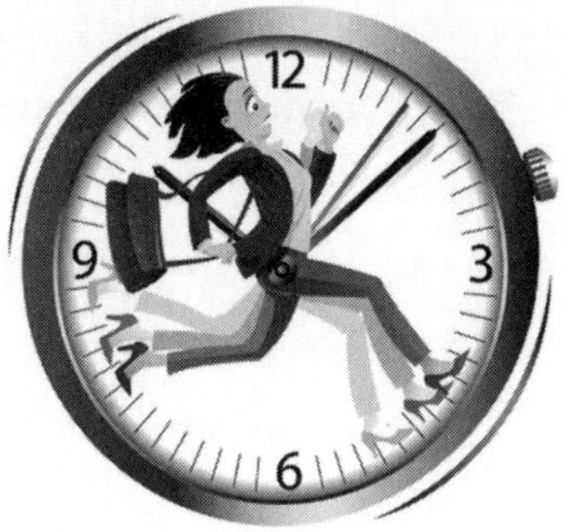

Introduction

Rushing Woman's Syndrome evolved out of my observation of a shift in women's health and behaviour over the past fourteen years. Never before in my work have I witnessed so many females in a mad rush to do everything and be all things to all people. Never before have I seen the extent of reproductive system problems that I now see. Women are wired. Many of them are tired too. Tired yet wired. And this relentless urgency, this perception that there is not enough time, combined with a to-do list that is never all crossed off, is having such significant health consequences for women that I had to write a book about it.

The perceived need to rush, whether a woman displays it on the outside or keeps it under wraps, is changing the face of women's health as we know it in such a detrimental way. Sex hormone-based health problems such as polycystic ovarian syndrome

(PCOS), endometriosis, infertility, and debilitating menopauses, not to mention exhaustion, have never been greater, and the role of stress in this is undeniable when you look at both the body's chemistry and the scientific research.

But I don't just care about the what… the imbalanced hormones, the burnt out adrenal glands from the long-term overproduction of stress hormones, the sluggish thyroid glands, and the impact that all of this has on us as well as the people around us… I care about the why just as much if not more; for it is the why that allows for sustained change. Why are women behaving and thinking in ways that are leading to this significant, downward spiral in their health? The answer lies in our biochemistry and our belief systems.

Once you understand what is really going on, you will see that the swing between rushing and not rushing is code for your beliefs and your behaviour is the outermost expression of those beliefs. For unless you question the beliefs upon which your actions are based, the actions will continue.

When you perceive that life is challenging, regardless of the circumstances, no matter how big or how small the challenges, how life threatening or not your problems are, to you the challenges are significant. I like to say "as with small things so with big things" meaning that how we handle the small stuff in life can also be how we respond to the big things in life.

Our body cannot keep up with the rate of change the world now asks of it and it is imperative that we understand this and take steps in our lives to create periods of down time, time in days, weeks, or months when we can truly rest. Just as we can't go without sleep for too long, your psyche cannot push on for too long without some quality downtime. If it does science is teaching us, and of course our intuition tells us, there will be consequences.

All species on the planet evolve every time they reproduce. The idea is that each new generation will be better equipped to cope with the prevailing conditions, the environment. Our challenge is that our surroundings are changing at a rate never before witnessed in human evolution. When I talk about evolution, I'm not talking about human evolution in the sense of biblical "creation" versus Darwinian "evolution." Instead I simply want you to consider what we are asking of our bodies.

Human beings have been on Earth for between 150,000 and 200,000 years. We evolved slowly and steadily over time, and, as nomads, we lived off the land that surrounded us as we moved. We were hunters and gatherers and only the seasons, the climate, and the weather conditions influenced our food choices and what we needed to do in a day. Humans ate fresh food precisely the way it came from nature and there were tasks to do to meet needs for survival. The diet was based primarily on green leaves, and other more concentrated foods were added when the opportunity arose from hunting and gathering.

Approximately 7,500 to 10,000 years ago, humans started to stay in one place for longer periods of time, and very basic agricultural practices were established. This was the first time we grew crops and the first time in human history that we consumed the milk of other animals. This was also the first time that repetition became significant in the human diet as a result of not having to chase our food down and also having a supply of crops in the field. Our patterns of eating and living, however, were still based on nature's rhythms, our produce was seasonal and at the mercy of floods and droughts and "work" was only able to be done in daylight hours.

While change continued at a very gradual, steady pace, the chemistry of the body could keep up. The next most significant change to our lifestyles came during the nineteenth century because of the Industrial Revolution. Processes were mechanized, and people started to move in big numbers from the country to the cities. There was an enormous reliance on agriculture for food production as population numbers continued to grow, and a day's work now required less movement as people came off the land and worked in the newly developed factories. Standards of living started to vary based on where we lived and how much we earned.

Propel forward to today and review our time on the planet. The past two decades—which have included the birth of the Internet and the invention of cell phones—have unleashed the most rapid period of change in human history to date. Not that long ago, when you left the house to go shopping or take children to school or while you drove from home to work, you were unreachable. Now, not only do our cell phones ring but they ping with the arrival of emails and social media comments. The majority of women I know don't sit idle when the traffic lights are red... they check for a text, emails, or the latest news from their favourite social media portal. Once upon a time when the lights were red, we had to contemplate or notice the colour of the sky or feel grateful or listen to a great song on the radio. There was naturally, without effort, more soul food and down time in our lives.

Now many people eat "food" containing non-food ingredients out of packets because they are in such a hurry. Food has to be convenient for many people or it is not on their menu. And the faster the better. But there's a cost as somewhere inside you, you know, whether you choose to acknowledge it or not. You would have had to have had your head buried in the sand for the last twenty years to not know that your diet needs to be based on fresh foods and that most people need to eat far more vegetables than they currently do. It is not a lack of education that drives most people's poor food choices. It is their beliefs. But instead of exploring ways to change their beliefs most people think they need more knowledge. In some cases of course further education about food, nutrition, lifestyle choices, and well-being can be immensely beneficial. Yet from where I'm sitting, inspiration too is just as important—that uplifted feeling of wanting to take such good care of yourself—and so is unravelling your beliefs.

I observe people today, particularly at airports. People step aboard a moving walkway and instead of continuing to walk to speed up their arrival at their departure gate, they stop. They're exhausted and they haven't even left yet! Contraptions have been designed to get us there quicker, yet some of these things also don't support our health. Instead, they stop us from moving. Today people don't have to climb stairs, as there are elevators, escalators, and moving walkways. We don't even have to go to the store to buy our food, let alone go into the fields and harvest it or chase it with a spear. We can order it online and have someone deliver it. There is no judgment here. Just a tip of the iceberg observation of how quickly and significantly the world in which we live has changed. We are guinea pigs in so many areas. Never before has a group of people been exposed to pesticides for their entire life or had a device that is known to emit radiation so close to our brains on a regular basis. Never before have artificial sweeteners, colours, and preservatives been in our food for the entirety of our lifetimes. I am crossing every finger and toe and even my eyes in the hope that all of these things are safe. My instinct tells me they are not.

At a cellular level, we basically have the same human body as our ancestors. Every generation evolves ever so slightly to be better equipped to inhabit its environment. This rate of evolution, however, is nothing compared to the change of pace in our world. Our conscious, thinking minds may have developed to keep up with the times, so that we are able to email while we talk on our cell phone at the same time that we recall we must remember to order a cake for our child's birthday (notice I inferred buy rather than bake), but biochemically we are much the same as we were 150,000 years ago. Still the same, too, is our subconscious mind, which research suggests is one million times more powerful than our conscious mind. Your subconscious mind, the part of your mind that you cannot access with your thoughts, the part that makes your heart beat and your hair grow, and knows how to heal a cut without you having to tell it to do so… don't you think those processes alone are truly amazing? I do not believe that our nervous systems, which enormously affect every cell of our bodies, every hormonal system, every organ, every aspect of fat burning, and our perception of urgency, have been able to keep up with the rate of change that this time in human history demands of us.

Between our cell phones and email systems, our laptops and wireless modems, we are asking our bodies to go places they have never ever been before. Never have we had a "mail" system that was immediate, a communication system that makes us accessible 24/7… if we allow it. Never have we had too little time to prepare our own food. Never have we held phones to our ears or plugged earphones into our ear sockets so that even when we exercise, we are both simultaneously distracting ourselves and overstimulating ourselves. What we are yet to truly realise en masse in the Western world is that the seeming urgency and the pace at which we are living is a disaster for human health, in particular for our nervous system and our reproductive system.

We are so far removed from our origins that many people think any or all of the following are either a luxury not available to them or hippy la-la concepts that they don't value: to eat seasonally, walk barefoot at times and feel the earth beneath their feet, turn their cell phone off after a particular time at night, not reply to emails within three minutes of receiving them and have a day of rest each week... and yes that does mean a day of not even checking emails.

We seem to have lost touch with the guiding light of nature when it comes to not just our food but also our whole way of living. And in my opinion, Mother Nature knows best. Once, not so long ago, we treated colds with garlic and lemons. Now, we take a pill and race on because we can't afford the time off from work. People go on vacation for a week and do three weeks worth of work the week before they go, just to get their work done, and then when they get back, usually even more exhausted than when they left, they have to catch up on a week's worth of emails and whatever else wasn't covered in their absence. When you take a step back, we sound like we've lost our minds, don't we? Essentially, it takes awareness and a commitment to live another way, a way that is more supportive of health on every level. With whole foods we are better nourished, and remember that it is nutrients that keep us alive. With more free time our relationships are better nurtured and we tend to be happier and kinder to both ourselves and those around us.

Probably without realising it you now ask your glands and organs, your liver, your gall bladder, your kidneys, your adrenals, your thyroid, your ovaries, your uterus, your brain, and your digestive system to cope with your rush. There are, of course, consequences to this superfast pace of living, and this book is partly borne out of my observations and reflections, as well as the science behind what this period in our evolution is requiring of us and doing to us.

We are not wired to cope with constant pressure, perceived or real, nor are we equipped long-term to eat poor quality food and lead sedentary lifestyles, strapped to our computers, cell phones plugged into our ear sockets. As I said, this is the tip of a partially inglorious but incredibly fascinating iceberg and the women of the Western world need to know both what it is doing to us and why we may have become caught up in the rush. Awareness is the first step and some of the contents herein will likely be new information for you. But some of it is simply a reminder of what you already know.

In writing this book I have used numerous examples and real-life stories of rushing women from all walks of life, with a wide variety of backgrounds and personal circumstances. A common scenario I've described is one of a working heterosexual mother. However, there are a multitude of other scenarios involving work, life, sexual preference, relationship status, socioeconomic situations that may or may not include children. I tell stories to help get the message across and I just wanted you to know that sometimes I generalize and recount what I hear most often... which is just one side of the story after all.

I am aware that the men in this world are suffering from the rush as well. I witness it every day. But the male psyche is somewhat different from the female so I have chosen to concentrate on women for this book. That is certainly not because I don't care about our men nor do I believe that their health is not being compromised by pressure and stress. I simply wanted to thoroughly explore why women are in a hurry more than ever before, what the consequences of this are, and of course offer insights and strategies that have the potential to foster change.

There will only ever be twenty-four hours in a day. And how you spend your time is entirely your choice. Your perception of what you need to do in a day is influenced by both your biochemistry and your beliefs. And you are about to gain some brand new insights into both. Come with me on this journey and take your understanding of your health to a whole new level and most importantly utilize the strategies and rituals offered here to change your health future.

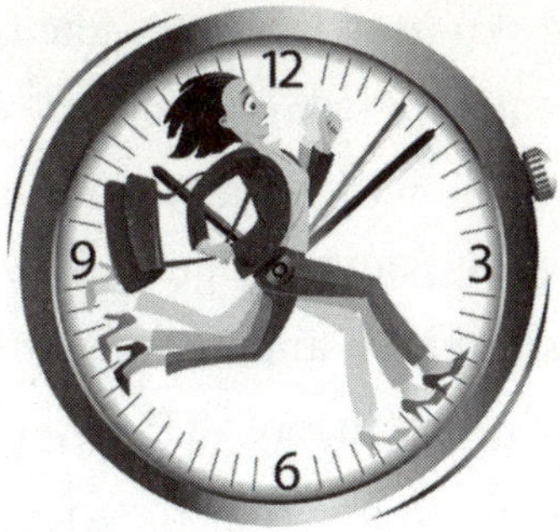

Chapter 1

What is Rushing Woman's Syndrome?

Rushing Woman's Syndrome (RWS) describes the biochemical effects of always being in a hurry and the health consequences that urgency elicits. It doesn't seem to matter if a woman has two things to do in her day or two hundred, she is in a pressing rush to do it all. She is wound up like a top, running herself ragged in a daily battle to keep up. There is always so much to do, and she very rarely feels like she wins, is in control and gets on top of things. In fact her deep desire to control even the smaller details of life can leave her feeling out of control, even of herself. Overwhelmed, at times she feels like she can't cope, whether she admits it out loud or keeps it all inside, adding to her wound up, knotted stomach. She is fortunate if her sex hormones are balanced. Most women in this state suffer terribly with their periods or don't bleed regularly, and women who go into menopause in this state usually find it debilitating.

The subgroup I lovingly call thyroid types cherish their coffee to the point that they feel they cannot live without it. They tell me that it clears the fog in their brain, gives them a tiny amount of energy (which is better than none), and that it keeps their bowels moving. They almost always tell me that coffee makes them happy. Thyroid types are less wired than others. It takes a lot of caffeine to amp them up. Thyroids are mostly tired. Beyond tired actually. It is in their bones. Whereas the majority of rushing women are wired and the tiredness is more debilitating in the later afternoon. Rushing Women typically get very weary in the late afternoon to early evening, but if they stay up after 10pm they often tell me that they get a second wind and it is then very hard to go to sleep until 2am.

The following is a checklist to help you identify if you are indeed a Rushing Woman.

A RUSHING WOMAN:

- Loves coffee to the point that she feels deprived if she cannot get her daily fix and she tells herself that she needs it for energy, to help her brain function, or so she can make her bowels move

- Answers "so busy" or "stressed" when you ask her how she is
- Has stress hormones, adrenalin and cortisol, pumping through her veins more often than she does not
- Has low progesterone
- Has problems with her periods which might look like polycystic ovarian syndrome, heavy, clotty periods, irregular periods, PMS, or a debilitating menopause
- Tends to crave sugar, particularly mid-afternoon or close to menstruation
- Feels overwhelmed often
- Has poor short-term memory
- Never feels like there are enough hours in the day
- Overreacts easily even if she doesn't display it outwardly
- Often feels tired but wired
- May have a thyroid gland that bounces between an underactive tendency and an overactive tendency

- Can't sit down as she will feel so guilty... unless she is beyond tired... then she will sit but she still feels guilty
- Sleeps too little
- Sometimes can't sleep restoratively
- Compromises sleep to get jobs done later at night
- Is irritable or, as I prefer to say, gritty
- Wants to speed when she drives, whether she needs to or not
- Wonders why everyone else drives so slow, whether they do or not
- Has no solitude, no time for self, and will tell you that's selfish or a luxury she could never have
- Has a to-do list that is never, ever all crossed off and this bothers her
- Feels a sense of panic easily
- Often has digestive system problems such as bloating or IBS
- Is so exhausted, particularly in the afternoon, a time when she is also more likely to feel like she cannot cope with her life... sugar, caffeine, or alcohol feel like the only options at this time

- Doesn't regularly notice the special moments she is part of… life feels mostly chaotic
- Laughs less than she used to
- Finds it difficult to relax without wine
- Has a mental fuzziness/haze/brain fog that she only notices is there when she has a random day when it is not
- Beats herself up for not being a good enough wife/mother/friend
- Is constantly looking for more ways to feel love or be praised, whether she can see this or not
- Feels anxious without her cell phone on her constantly… she can catch herself constantly pushing the refresh screen button thinking—"what if I miss an important text or phone call?" and takes her phone to the toilet for this reason
- Goes on holiday only to spend the majority of the time thinking she must unwind yet never actually resting… holidays simply become an extension of her usual life
- Tends to return from a break feeling even more exhausted than before she left

- Takes short and shallow breaths and can often become breathless; may sigh frequently
- Low appetite or, on the contrary, feels as though she could eat her arm off, particularly at night
- Can tend to blame others for adding to her workload or "stressing her out"—when a lot of the stress comes from her own internal pressures
- Whilst trying to achieve as much as possible in the day can catch herself checking emails in the bathroom, at traffic lights, or late at night
- Goes to guilt as a common emotional pattern
- Doesn't usually ask for help
- Can't say no easily and if she does… she feels guilty!

How many of the above statements do you relate to? To have a bit of fun with this, count up the number of statements you relate to and explore your level of rushing using the scale below!

0 = This book is not for you. But, before you put it aside, read on as it will more than likely relate to some of your friends!

1-4 = You are not a Rushing Woman. Instead, use this book to identify the areas of your endocrine system that may need some extra support. For example, if you experience PMS, apply the strategies suggested for that particular condition.

5-7 = You are well on your way to becoming a Rushing Woman! Apply the strategies suggested to support both your physical and emotional health and get your score down and level of well-being up!

7 or above = Hello Rushing Woman. It is a delight to meet you and to be able to assist you come down from the stress mountain.

THE PHYSICAL HEALTH OF A RUSHING WOMAN

There are a number of body systems involved in the rush. They are the:

- Nervous system
- Endocrine system which includes the:
    - Adrenal glands (where we make our stress hormones)
    - Ovaries
    - Thyroid gland
    - Pituitary gland, the master switch (housed inside the brain)
- Digestive system

Any or all of these systems may be affected by a

hurried lifestyle. When you address just one of these systems, you might feel somewhat better. However, if the mad rush continues, your overall health is likely to continue to suffer, and potentially decline. Helping you sort out your biochemistry is a big part of what this book is intended to do. In the next few chapters, you will learn not only how to identify which of your systems needs attention and particular care, but also what to do about them.

When your biochemistry is out of whack—for example, your sex hormones—it can be very difficult to change how you feel. You may suffer from a tendency to get stuck in feeling overwhelmed, have frequent meltdowns, or burst with angry explosions or all of the above. Your body constantly receives messages from the environment and from within the body itself about the chemicals (hormones) it needs to make and sorting these out can go a long way towards helping you slow down and not feel like everything had to be done yesterday.

The following is a piece I wrote for a national newspaper that seemed to ring a few bells for those who read it.

Rushing Woman's Syndrome

Take a deep breath and come on a journey of food and hormones, thoughts and perceptions, energy and vitality, with me.

Naturally there are variations in the details of what I am about to describe but I think you'll get the gist...

A typical pattern of food intake that I witness regularly is this: you get up in the morning, inhale some sort of processed breakfast cereal, and race out the door to work. Your blood sugar soars, and your pancreas subsequently releases a surge of insulin. Welcome to fat storage situation number one of your day. You take shallow breaths all morning due to the perceived pressures and deadlines in your day and your to-do list is never all ticked off. After your peak in blood sugar from your breakfast, by mid-morning, your blood sugar plummets, and concentration levels are waning. You are relieved when you look at your watch at 10:30am. You have not achieved an awful lot up until now in your day other than trying to get on top of emails that you actually never seem to get on top of, but at least 10:30am means morning tea time, an opportunity to get away from your desk, either with colleagues or by yourself, and head to the nearest coffee cart or café.

You justify your desire, and subsequent purchase of a muffin, along with your large double shot skinny milk latte, by telling yourself that you have a big day ahead and you'll probably go to the gym later anyway. Welcome to fat storage situation number two of your day, thanks to your coffee and muffin. You return to your desk and push on with some work, but, after about one or two hours, you are fidgety again and want lunch. Your blood sugar has come down from its high brought on by your mid-morning snack. You look at your watch again... thank goodness it is lunch time! And out you go for lunch.

You know you feel better in your tummy on days when you don't eat bread for lunch, but you tell yourself that you are busy and you need to be quick. A sandwich, bagel, or a roll is always quick and easy. You inhale it. Then you want something sweet. Hmmm. Chocolate? No, not yet. Fruit. OK, good choice, you think. And, on the inside, your blood sugar and subsequently your insulin level surge again (fat storage situation number three for the day). Within half an hour, you feel utterly exhausted, probably bloated, and you are berating yourself because you feel fat. You are, in fact, simply bloated, but your discomfort and the wind building in your tummy, coupled with your "fat" abdomen make you feel gross. You work in an open plan office, so you are conscious of hanging on to that wind in case it has an odour. And so even though your colleagues may be (unknowingly) grateful, the bloating and hence the size of your tummy increases over the afternoon.

The psychological process that goes

on in your head, particularly if you are a woman, after lunch when you reflect on what you have consumed that morning, is incredibly detrimental to your health and your cortisol levels and, hence, your waistline. You feel like all you did was eat all morning and sit on your bottom. You think about the dress you were planning to fit into to wear to an event three weeks from now. Even though all you have done is eat breakfast, a muffin, a coffee, and a roll, in that moment, you believe that your thighs are extra wobbly this afternoon, that you will never fit into that dress, and even though you were thinking you would go to the gym that evening, having not achieved very much over your morning, you know you will stay back at work and not go. You think about the gym membership that cost you a bomb and that you haven't used for the last three months, and you feel useless. You think again about the "massive" (as perceived by you), amounts of food you have eaten that day so far, and you hate yourself and your swollen abdomen. Then! Light bulb! A thought that suddenly makes you feel better flashes into your mind. You suddenly feel back in control. What was that thought? There at your desk in this bloated abdomen post-lunch state, you decide that you won't eat afternoon tea! You feel better immediately because you have found a way out of your perceived eating frenzy and expanding (bloated) waistline. Oh the joys for a frantic female mind with body concerns.

Yet your blood sugar and insulin picture over your morning resembled a roller coaster, and just because you have decided that you are not going to eat afternoon tea, how do you expect your blood sugar to be any different from the way it was in the morning? The answer is it won't be. By 3:00 to 4:00pm, your blood sugar has plummeted again, and you feel exhausted. The momentary elation from your "no afternoon tea" thought after lunch has vaporised and you are now "starving" to the point that you could eat your arm off. Your blood sugar is rock bottom. So, instinctively, what type of food do you think your body will desperately want you to eat in this situation? You guessed it. Sugar. Almost nothing raises your blood sugar faster, and your biochemical drive for survival knows it.

But you said you wouldn't eat afternoon tea! And now you feel so desperate for it, nothing is going to stand in your way. But if you give in and you eat something, when you said you wouldn't, what emotion do you feel? Guilt. And what stress hormone do you think guilt drives your body to make? Cortisol, which, when produced in excess, is another fat storage hormone. What a vicious and exhausting cycle. Oh yes, did I mention you feel exhausted?

So you give in and you eat whatever sweet fix you can lay your hands on. Some women will placate the need for food at this time and get their second coffee for the day. It is highly unlikely that a black coffee would hit the spot at this time of day; it almost always has to be milky... you'll tell yourself need "substance"! Those who choose the coffee partially feel good because they didn't give in and eat, but then these people "know" in the back of their mind that extra coffees in their day are not ideal for them either. New clients express precisely this to me every day of my working life. But they console themselves with, "at least I didn't eat."

Those who do eat feel momentarily better with yet another elevation in blood sugar and consequently insulin. Hello fat storage situation number four for the day. And then the self-directed cruel statements silently begin. "You are hopeless. You have no willpower. Look at your stomach." It is the "will I, won't I, I said I wouldn't, but I did" (BID) syndrome, often a key catchphrase for Rushing Women. And, from that headspace, you lament from your desk at 6:30pm, when you are still there trying to get on top of the work you didn't do that day because you were so busy thinking about food and exercise and dresses and your stomach and not passing wind, that you can't go to the gym now because it is already 6:30pm. You still have more work to do, and if you work until 7:15pm, well there is no food at home so you will have to go to the supermarket, and, if you go to the supermarket, it will then be 8pm before you get home and then you still have to chop the vegetables, and that takes aaaaages, and then you still have to cook, eat, and clean up, and so it will be at least 11:30pm before you are finished doing all of that, and you probably need to do more work at home that night. But you have to wash your hair in the morning and then straighten it and so you need to get up earlier to do that... and then you get up and do it all over again, and you wonder why you can't lose weight when you don't eat "that badly" and why you are always so exhausted. You can see it is biochemical and it is psychological. And of course, if you then throw sleep deprivation into that mix... what a cocktail! This powerful combination has the potential to promote fat storage rather than accessing fat to burn for energy and that drive surges and plummets of energy and happiness.

This is a pattern common to so many women. Although I may have exaggerated some of the details of the scenario above (or not really!) and there are many variations to what I have described which may include children, partners, parents, friends, and work not based in an office, I meet women of all ages who live like this day after day after day. There may or may not be big, traumatic stresses going on, but there is a daily, relentless juggling act that never ends. It is typical of adults between the ages of twenty-five and sixty-five, although it tends to be far more prominent in those between the ages of thirty and fifty-five. It often stems from a desire to be all things to all people, from being a "pleaser," behaviour that was probably rewarded in childhood. It makes people like you, and you feel good assisting and being there for others. You find it hard to put yourself first and on the odd occasion you do, a nagging guilt tends to arise. You are exhausted and the only time you don't feel that way is when you are living on adrenalin.

The cocktail of hormones being made in the BID and the RW syndromes mostly involves cortisol and insulin. This disastrous cocktail in turn interferes with progesterone production, so estrogen dominance prevails, giving you heavy, clotty periods and PMS. This downregulates thyroid function, so you drink coffee, wine, or both, to speed up and cool down respectively each day, and your liver gets a regular thumping, and still no one eats enough green vegetables. Throw in some emotional confusion and chaos and you have what I call Rushing Woman's Syndrome.

So on the one hand, one way to begin to solve this health picture is through food, through dietary change that evens out your blood glucose and hence your insulin production. Yet on the other hand, you can also see that it is not only about the food. Because that rushing feeling, even when, if you paused, you would know in your heart that there is no need to rush, as well as your unconscious need to please and your mean self-talk... these tend to be the common emotional factors that can lead us to make poor food and beverage choices. It is time to slow down precious people.

~~~~~~~~~~~~~~~~~~~~~~~

THE EMOTIONAL HEALTH OF A RUSHING WOMAN

There is far more to the Rushing Woman than simply her hormones being out of balance. You haven't always been like this. You certainly weren't born in this state. The rush is learned.

You can most likely recall a time in your life when everything somehow seemed simpler, and you may find yourself craving this feeling again. Yet when you look at how you might alter your current life, women often feel helpless to change anything because things seem intertwined and therefore complicated. For example, "if I do what I really want to which is to work less and spend more time with the children, we
~~~~~~~~~~~~~~~~~~~~~~~

can't make the mortgage repayments and pay our other bills so I can't go part time. But I'm exhausted and yet I'm aware my husband is under just as much pressure. And if I reduce my paid work he will feel even more financial pressure and I worry about his health, for his sake and of course the children's, and so it is just easier if I keep doing everything." Do you know how many times I've heard versions of this sentiment? Thousands. And I have to admit there is a part of me that wants to tell people to sell their house, buy something cheaper, spend less, want less from a material perspective, reduce their mortgage because I am yet to experience a house that goes even close to outweighing the importance of human health. From what I have observed and also experienced personally, no house is worth it. Sure this is only one scenario but I simply wanted to demonstrate how our desire to take better care of ourselves can sometimes feel like an impossible dream. But every knotted piece of string has two ends. Find one of them and ask for help to unravel it if you cannot see the way forward yourself.

Certainly the present pace of life has catapulted us into a new realm with unique pressures and an unprecedented intensity. Sure, our mothers and grandmothers didn't have cell phones and emails and more office work to attend to after the kitchen was clean and the washing and ironing were put away... yes times have changed. Our mothers had their own way of dealing with the pressures they felt. They may have spent money, if they had it, or eaten too much. Some of them possibly drank too much alcohol and some might have been outwardly content yet very worried on the inside. Most females have always been scared about "getting into trouble" or "letting others down." It is just that now, with technology, the push, push, push and the rush, rush, rush, there is an added, and I believe even more damaging to our health, road for a significant emotional pattern to be expressed, a pattern that is specifically feminine. And our nervous systems, our reproductive systems, and our digestive systems are suffering like never before as a result of it. What is it? What is this emotional pattern I'm claiming has been around for longer than the rush—that the rush has brought closer to the surface, more out into the open—for a health professional like me to observe?

THE WHY

This is a big bold statement: Rushing Woman's Syndrome comes from your relentless pursuit to never feel rejected.

Your deepest need to never feel rejected was set up when you were a little girl. It happens to more girls that it does not. From a look on your mother's face, the way your parents might have cut you off with their impatient tones when you had something important to say, or your father's odd behaviour when he'd had too much to drink... from any, or all, of these scenarios, or another that is particular to you, you created a meaning that your parents didn't love you and that you had to be someone you were not to have them love you. And you've spent the rest of your life, on some level, doing absolutely everything you can to never, ever, ever feel that way (shut out, unloved, ostracized, abandoned, neglected) again. So you please people. Anyone and everyone. You can't sleep if you are worried you've upset someone. And if you particularly, desparately have to please your intimate partner (and if he is male or she has a masculine essence), you have a stronger connection to avoiding rejection set up by interactions with your father than your mother. Whereas if your partner comes way down your list in your "urgency to please" behaviour, your fear of rejection from the masculine was most likely outweighed by that set up by your feminine role model, most often your mother.

Many rushing women despise conflict. They will do anything to avoid it, including, "alter the truth." One of her mottos is "keep the peace." I am stunned at the number of women, and women who earn their own money, who lie to their husbands about what they spend. Often when I catch up with one of my rather entertaining friends, she tells me how she went shopping on the weekend and bought boots, a scarf, and a handbag she'd been eying off for ages… and she scuffed both the boots and the bag before she wore/used them for the first time so her husband wouldn't notice that they were new and ask what they cost. Another friend used a marker to change the price on the ticket of a top she bought once she was home so it looked like the top was discounted in the store. When I asked what would happen if he found out that she'd paid full price for the top she said "I'd get into trouble"… this from a grown woman who works hard running her own business. Start to reflect already on your own behaviours. You may not change the price of things but there are potentially other things you do to keep the peace.

Because of the stress, both physical… from low nutrient-density diets, lack of sleep, too many foods and drinks that make it hard for the liver to work optimally and efficiently, and emotional… from the relentless urgency to please and avoid rejection, our adrenal glands, the place in the body where our stress hormones are made, are often in overdrive. And when our stress hormones are consistently elevated, our sex hormone balance is massively disrupted, concepts explored in detail later in the book. All you need to know right now is that you can unravel this. That's why I've written this book. It is a physical, emotional, and spiritual journey that can be, at times, challenging and confronting, yet utterly magnificent, enlightening, and, ultimately, one that reminds you that the peace you seek in within you.

There is a concept in emergency medicine called triage, where patients are assigned a degree of urgency based on how quickly their wounds need treating. And I've decided this is what women do all day long. Our daily existence can involve the constant assessment of who needs our attention the most... children, husband, work, best friend, mother, kind neighbour, not-so-kind neighbour, unwell friend, overflowing rubbish bin... We tend to leave ourselves off this list, yet if I were to ask the majority of women if they believe they have omitted themselves because they are selfless, most reply with an emphatic "No! I simply don't have time." If we don't have time for ourselves, soon we'll have nothing left to give.

When I was almost finished writing *Rushing Woman's Syndrome*, a friend told me I needed to see the film *I Don't Know How She Does It*. Having been in hibernation, writing mode for quite a while,

I didn't even know about it or that the film is based on a book by the brilliant Allison Pearson. Loving nothing better than a great read, I later came across a book of the same name in my local book shop and made the link. So of course I grabbed it. I tend to love the detail the written word offers more than the way nuances are depicted in movies, so I was determined to read the book before I see the film. But to get this manuscript done by its deadline, I could not stop to read or I would not come back to my computer for days!!! BUT! Being the bookworm I am, I opened the book and read a random page, just one little page… and it communicated a message so beautifully that I share it with you as it expresses how most women feel that their rush and the juggling act will never be over and that their tasks will never be done.

> Stress eczema the nurse at work called it. "Can you think of any way to relieve some of the pressures in your life Kate?" Oh let's see now: a brain transplant, a Lottery win, my husband being reprogrammed to figure out that things left at the bottom of the stairs usually need to be carried to the top of the stairs.

It is easy to get caught up in a story you tell yourself about how hard/busy/tough/neverending/overwhelming… your life is. I know. I've been there too. And it is so easy to blame the people around you. You cannot change them. You can only change yourself. And if you pause and focus on this precise moment, there is nothing but peace and beauty, and that can permeate your entire existence if that is what you want. It is always there, always available, waiting for you to notice.

I witnessed a friend recently throw away an opportunity to be present when I commented on how precious her three children's clothes looked hanging on the staircase railing, all pressed and tiny and ready for school the next day. And their little shoes were lined up beneath each outfit. When I commented to my friend, the children's mother, on what a sweet sight it was, and she (bless her in her exhaustion) rolled her eyes and said it is Groundhog Day to her. In an instant she saw what she had done... washed over a moment in time, missed soaking up the soul-nourishing sight at the bottom of the stairs, for her mind had jumped ahead to what tomorrow would, in her mind be—another morning of feeling beyond exhaustion and of chaos and demands on her time and energy. Yet the beauty of life and the beauties expelled by the lives we helped create is there to behold if we can BE in the moment, rather than always being ahead of it. Yes, we have to plan and organize, of course we do. But my goodness the feelings of stress are so much less when we have moments of noticing and soaking up the immense beauty around us. And the stress is so much less if we invest in ourselves, whatever that looks like for you. Going to your local café and reading a magazine, sitting outside where you live and letting the sun warm your back, with only the birds to keep you company, starting the day with qi gong and a walk. Part of what I will encourage you to do, to shift your perception that there is never enough time, involves creating a spaciousness in your life. And there are many ways to create this as you will see.

I spoke at a lunch with a friend of mine who is a psychologist with a great wit. He asked the audience of women to describe what romance meant to them. The majority of the women in the room responded with comments such as "when he vacuums the floor" and "when he takes the garbage out without being asked." Very few responded with what they may have been more likely to say at the beginning of a courtship such as "calling me outside to share a sunset," "a bunch of flowers for no reason" and "my husband's face lighting up when he sees me." And what struck me, with the majority of comments being focused on helping around the house, was how time-poor women perceive themselves to be. If taking out the garbage has become romance, you feel you have too much on your plate to handle! There would not have been a woman in the room who married her husband for his vacuuming skills! Yet this is what many women have come to perceive as romance. I am not denying for one second that receiving help makes an enormous difference to how we feel and that teamwork in a marriage is vital. What I am saying is that when taking out the garbage has become how you want romance demonstrated to you, you are overwhelmed with your to-do list, and it is time for a new perspective.

Not so long ago, women began doing what had historically been their father's jobs, while they maintained their mother's responsibilities. What has transpired for many women is a frantic double shift. Women do the same jobs now as men and they do them equally well. But all the time, women are carrying around information that won't seem to leave them alone. To paraphrase Allison Pearson, the inside of a woman's head is akin to Heathrow airport. "Vaccinations (to jab or not to jab), reading programs, shoe sizes of each family member, best friend's marital woes and what to do about them, contraception, would the kids be better off in childcare, would the kids be better off at home, grocery items, changed my mind about that guy I met last week... must text him, the six reports that were due to the client an hour ago, need to remind the nanny to stop washing whites with colours, must straighten my hair tonight, what time is the courier coming?" My friend Amanda calls them "first world problems." All of this information just circles in our heads awaiting further instruction from air traffic control. If women didn't bring all that they do safely in to land, the whole world would fall apart. Instead, the health of women is coming undone in a way that is preventable.

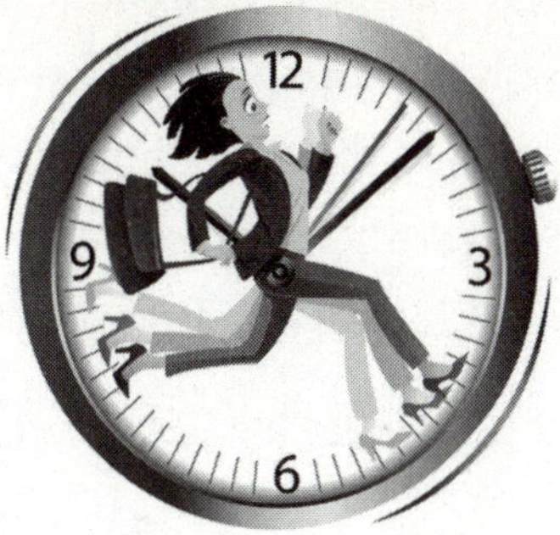

Chapter 2
The Nervous System: its role in the rush

When it comes to your health and your degree of calm, one body system stands out above all others… your nervous system.

The nervous system is comprised of various body parts including your brain, your spinal cord, and the nerves that connect your brain to every organ of your body. There are several parts to your nervous system which include the Central Nervous System (CNS) and the Autonomic Nervous System (ANS). The ANS has two branches known as the Sympathetic Nervous System (SNS) and the Parasympathetic Nervous System (PNS). Rather than worrying about remembering all of these long-winded names, just know that the SNS drives the "fight or flight" response, while the

PNS promotes the “rest and digest” also known as the “rest and repair” response. This is diagrammatically represented in the following figure.

CNS (under conscious control)

ANS (under subconscious control)

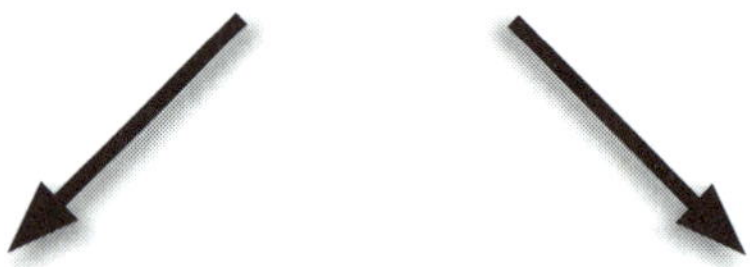

SNS (fight or flight)

PNS (rest and digest)

Different Parts of the Nervous System: *The CNS and ANS are controlled differently, while the SNS and the PNS are branches of the ANS.*

Your CNS is governed by your conscious mind; that is, you control it with your thoughts. For example, if you want to write, you choose to pick up a pen and write. If you choose to walk, you control the direction in which and the pace at which you travel. You choose it. Your ANS, however, is controlled by your subconscious mind. In other words you are *unable* to access it with your thoughts. Your ANS governs how quickly your heart beats, how fast your hair and nails grow; rates over which you have no control. You cannot suddenly wake up and remember that you are going to a party on Saturday night and think that it would be fun to turn up with hair down to your waist… it doesn't work like that. Your hair will grow to your waist (if that's what you want!) in its own sweet time. You have no say in it.

It is the ANS that is so enormously affected by rushing. And you are also enormously affected by the way your ANS responds to what you may not even realise you think about or perceive. Before we proceed further in understanding the role of the nervous system in our health when it comes to rushing, I first want to share with you the role the nervous system plays in the human body using fat as its fuel, particularly given that body fat that won't shift can be a source of frustration and stress for many women and make them hurry around even more. When I share this information with audiences when I speak live, one of the joys in my life is witnessing their eyes light up with understanding and their hearts open to a whole new realm of possibility when it comes to their weight, their health, and how they feel and function every day, one that has zero to do with calories. So here you go…

THE NERVOUS SYSTEM AND BODY FAT

In any given moment the human body is making a decision about which fuel to use based on the information it is receiving. The only two fuels for the human body are glucose ("sugar") and fat. You don't use protein for fuel. The body breaks protein down into amino acids which are then converted into glucose so the body can use that glucose as fuel (energy). The body requires energy for everything it does, from walking to sleeping and from laughing to blinking; it all requires fuel.

Adrenalin, one of the stress hormones the body makes easily and often regularly in the modern world, communicates to every cell of your body that your life is in danger and it prepares you to fight or flee. However, you may be making adrenalin simply because you have to make a phone call that you'd rather not make or perhaps because you've gulped down three coffees already today. The stress for most people in the Western world today is psychological rather than physical.

The branch of the nervous system that is activated with stress of any type is the sympathetic nervous system, which has an intimate relationship with adrenalin. If the body's perception is that it needs to escape from impending danger, whether your thinking mind is telling you so or not, you need a fast-burning fuel available to you to do that. Your body thinks it has to get out of there and get out of there fast! So what fuel do you think your body will choose when it needs to flee, to get out of "danger" fast? Remember its only choice is to either burn sugar or fat... in this scenario, it will choose sugar every time. The body thinks it has to in order to save our life and we are all about survival. The body doesn't feel "safe" enough to use fat as its fuel in this fight or flight state because fat offers us a steady, slow release form of energy. We can burn fat effectively in a PNS-dominant state because the body perceives it is safe when the PNS is activated. Yet, the PNS can never be the dominant arm of the ANS, it can never steer the ship, while the body perceives there may be a threat to your life.

We have glucose stored in our muscles and liver in a form called glycogen, and these stores are mobilized whenever our body gets the message that it needs energy to fight or run, if there is not enough to fuel our escape left in our blood from our last meal. This mobilization of glycogen out of the muscles due to stress can, over time, impact the function and appearance of our muscles, including allowing the onset of cellulite, particularly at the top of a woman's legs.

I believe that one of the most enormous health challenges of modern times is that the body can constantly be on the receiving end of the fight or flight message. There are so many factors, internal and external to us, that drive this response within us (explored in a moment) that we have to begin to actively choose not to go there, not to get caught up in the rush, and take steps in our daily lives to allow our nervous system to have some balance.

THE NERVOUS SYSTEM IN BODY FAT LOSS AND ANXIETY

The following is an extract from my book *Accidentally Overweight* explaining the role of the nervous system in fat loss and anxiety.

> ### *THE NERVOUS SYSTEM*
>
> The function of our nervous system is influenced by the way we move and exercise, the food we eat, the thoughts we think and our subconscious responses to our interactions and the life around us. Most people believe that in order to become healthy they must lose some weight. I believe the opposite is true; in order to lose weight, we must become healthy, and I approach weight loss in this way. As I've described using science, emotion, and real-life stories throughout *Accidentally Overweight*, I have known thousands of people who subsist off very little, exercise rampantly, but never get anywhere when it comes to fat loss.
>
> How else can we approach this? And how does this lifestyle create what I lov-

ingly call the Rushing Woman Syndrome? For some, the RW Syndrome is at the heart of them becoming *Accidentally Overweight*. Don't get me wrong—some women I meet living the RW Syndrome life are slim. But their nervous systems are usually a wreck, too, and nervous system imbalance takes a significant toll on our health and usually our relationships.

To understand this, we need to explore how the autonomic nervous system (ANS) works. The autonomic nervous system "runs" our body behind the scenes, and it is not under our conscious control. It regulates our heart rate, our respiration rate, our temperature control, and our immune and hormonal systems while we carry on with life. Don't you think it is miraculous that if you cut yourself the wound just heals? Don't you think it is amazing that you swallow food and your digestive system extracts the nutrients to nourish you so you can stay alive? The human body is extraordinary, and that's an understatement.

There are three parts to the autonomic nervous system. They are the sympathetic nervous system (SNS), the parasympathetic nervous system (PNS), and the enteric nervous system (ENS). I'm going to focus on the sympathetic nervous system, the "fight or flight" system, and the parasympathetic nervous system, the "rest and repair" system, and their interaction.

In general, the SNS and the PNS have opposite functions. When we are under stress, the SNS raises our heart rate, increases our respiratory rate, releases cortisol, and shunts blood away from the digestive tract to the muscles so that we can run away from or fight whatever is threatening us. If organ systems in the body are unhealthy and therefore stressed themselves, or if we are mentally or emotionally stressed, that increases the sympathetic load as well. The SNS by its very nature is catabolic, meaning that it breaks down muscle tissue due to the increased amounts of secreted cortisol. High-intensity exercise is also sympathetic in nature; the heart rate goes up, as does respiration and body temperature, and cortisol is released into the blood. And we know what cortisol does to body fat and the hormonal changes it initiates. Once the threat is dealt with (is it ever dealt with in the modern world?), the PNS slows our heart rate and respiration, brings the blood back to the digestive tract so that we can digest our food and be well nourished, works on repairing any tissues that have been damaged in our "battle," and allows libido to be restored. Your survival instinct can't have you thinking about sex when your body believes that your life is being threatened! The PNS is able to do its wonderful work overnight, provided we go to bed early enough, because cortisol naturally starts to rise at around 2:00am. The SNS and the PNS are designed to balance each other, and, in those people who have a well-balanced nervous system, high-intensity exercise will lead to fat loss because the parasympathetic rest time between work-outs is when muscle tissue is built.

It is likely that people who are unable to lose fat by doing regular high-intensity exercise have a dominant SNS and, as a result, an inhibited PNS. In situations like this, there is too much systemic "stress" coming from somewhere, and therefore adding high-intensity exercise is counter-productive, since it adds to an individual's sympathetic load, exacerbating the nervous system imbalance. This is one of the reasons we have to get our heads around "it's not about the calories" when it comes to weight loss. If "burning" more of them has not solved your body-fat challenge up until now, it is not suddenly going to start until some other work is done.

Anxiety is incredibly common today, often as a result of relationship challenges, a fixation on weight loss, financial stress, a poor diet and its consequences, or concerns about health. Yet, a person may be in sympathetic overload and still not even mention feeling anxious or stressed! Alarmingly, *not* living this way is becoming the exception.

Reducing the sympathetic load is essential to fat loss if the SNS is dominant. Movement is still important, but it is best approached from a different angle and with a different attitude. Far more effective exercise for SNS-dominant people is what I call the more "yin" (gentle, feminine, as opposed to "yang," masculine, go go go) forms of exercise, such as tai chi, qi gong, restorative yoga, or any exercise that is done slowly and while being conscious of the breath. These types of exercise significantly assist in increasing PNS activity, which helps balance the ANS. Once the body is better balanced and healthier, body fat is readily burnt.

I hope that it is quite clear that although this book (*Accidentally Overweight*) is about solving your weight loss puzzle, I am also gently unfolding information that might open your eyes and your heart to the concept that weight loss involves the superb interaction of many biochemical systems, and that your thoughts, beliefs, and perceptions are just as powerful, if not more powerful, than the food you eat.

~~~~~~~~~~~~~~~~~~~~~~~~

SYMPATHETIC NERVOUS SYSTEM DOMINANCE

The majority of women I see in my practice, and even those I meet on the street, are SNS dominant. Their perception of what they have to do in a day is
~~~~~~~~~~~~~~~~~~~~~~~~

overwhelming to them. They have usually elevated their adrenalin production and pushed themselves further into SNS dominance with caffeine over the morning as well. Even the calmest, most grounded woman will be fizzing, on the inside at least, with a few coffees under her belt for the day... for some even one caffeinated beverage is enough to amp them up so significantly that they overreact to the smallest thing and both fat burning and calm are blocked. The calming, anti-anxiety sex hormone progesterone is typically low due to too much cortisol (stress hormone) and too much estrogen (from food, the environment, and from liver recycling, which is often the result of the regular reliance on alcohol to "relax" in the evenings after being so amped up during the day... more on this in a moment) and as a result the mad rush feelings and the overreaction to things tends to be worse in the lead up to menstruation. Throw in some sugary snacks and perhaps more caffeine when the afternoon exhaustion kicks in, and you have a cocktail of behaviours aimed at reducing stress that are in fact adding a significant level of stress to your body.

On top of the physical stressors, are the emotional responses that do not serve us and keep us in an SNS dominant state. As children, these emotional patterns probably served a purpose of protection but now as adults they are often detrimental to our mental and therefore our physical health, and often our personal growth. I've listed a few of the most common emotional patterns I observe in rushing women below.

EXHAUSTING EMOTIONAL PATTERNS THAT CONTRIBUTE TO SNS DOMINANCE

An inability to say no

I have heard it countless times from female clients and friends… I don't know how to say no. There are many times in our lives when we want to say no but instead we say yes, usually to please other people and keep the peace. We want others to like us and we behave as if saying no sometimes will either lead them to believe that we don't like them or that they will think we are a terrible person. And when we spell it out on paper like this, you can see how crazy it is! A client recently shared a great example of this pattern with me. She was scheduled to go into the hospital to have a baby and she had one day of solitude planned, the day before she was to give (caesarian) birth. Her older children were going to be at school and she simply wanted a peaceful day at home by herself to reflect and rest and be. So when her neighbour asked if my client could look after her sick child for a few hours while she went to a meeting, my client said yes… and begrudged her neighbour for asking. Yet if she had simply explained to her neighbour her plans for the day, it would have given her neighbour an opportunity to explore other options. It is time to stop giving up what you want to keep the peace. Sure it is lovely to give. Contributing to the world and those around you is a fundamental need for humans... contribution helps give our lives meaning. Yet when we do it at our own expense and say yes when secretly we wish we'd said no, it doesn't serve anybody.

This pattern, the inability to say no, is a major drain on our energy, not to mention our time. It revs our stress response, driving us in to, or holding us in SNS dominance. And our adrenal glands, which release the stress hormones, can also be significantly impacted upon over time. It is crucial to learn to say no. However, knowing that this will help your health is usually not enough to promote change. You will tell yourself you need to say no far more often than you currently do, yet your subconscious drive to avoid pain (the perceived loss of love from those asking things of you) will usually lead you back to being a yes girl. We explore the psychology of this in a later chapter.

Seeking acceptance, approval, appreciation, and love

Another way the above words could be phrased

is "seeking to avoid rejection" or "to avoid being ostracized." When we constantly aim to prove our worth to the people in our lives or the people we meet, it is exhausting and adds another layer of stress to busy lives. However, when I'm working with an individual, what I've noticed is that at first, they usually can't reconcile their behaviour with wanting to fit in and be accepted. And then the penny drops... you can see it on someone's face, and the best way I can describe the expression is one of relief. And they look lighter, more free somehow. For the penny to drop, you often have to look down upon a situation in your own life as if you were an angel watching from above. Only you look down upon yourself and sometimes, with a curious attitude rather than any form of judgement or preconceived ideas about what might going on, you see the situation as it really is and that you simply said or did what you did, to be accepted, approved of, appreciated and ultimately loved. And there is nothing wrong with that. I only want to make you aware of what drives you, so that if that behaviour also harms you in some way, for example stresses you out and keeps you in SNS dominance, you have the power to change it. When you don't know why you do the things you do, when you just know that you always seem to end up doing things you don't want to do, or perhaps you feel used and unappreciated and unhappy, you are lost without a map. Looking down upon your precious self helps you see your path out.

Not putting you first

On an aeroplane the safety video always suggests you put on your own oxygen mask first before helping others, the premise behind which is that if you pass out you will not be able to assist others. It is very easy to pay lip service to this concept and another story entirely to actually act on it. When you go to meditate or practice yoga or go to a café to read your favourite magazine, you are taking care of you and nurturing your soul, and this helps everyone around you. Typically, we are able to behave in a much calmer and kinder manner when we have put some runs on our own board and created a sense of spaciousness in our lives. When people tell me they have no time, of course I know they are busy. What I also know is that they have no space in their mind to fit another task, another thing to remember. It is headspace women need, and only you can give yourself that. Start to incorporate relaxation rituals into your everyday life. Don't wait until you actually feel stressed.

A girlfriend of mine had started to dread picking her five children up from school. Aged between nine and seventeen, she said "every day, it was chaos and the boys are at that age where they smell after school and it was just so loud for the twenty-minute drive home that I'd feel so stressed by the time we got there, I'd end up screaming at them on a daily basis. I couldn't cope and yet I felt like such a dreadful mother for yelling at them. One day, to prepare myself for the school pickup, I listened to spa music while I drove and so it was on when the older children got into the car. After initially teasing me about my taste in music and making a few "om" noises, we had the calmest drive home we'd had since they hit puberty. So now that's part of my daily ritual. It doesn't always completely negate the chaos but it's certainly much less and I, too, am different. I'm not drowning now. I respond to them differently, from a much more centred space."

Guilt

Guilt is such a futile emotion. What leads you to feel guilty? Most often it is your perception that you have let someone else down. Yet when you pause to think about that, it is simply a story you are telling yourself. The reality is that it is not physically possible to let another human being down. If you do or say something, it is the other person's choice *entirely* whether they feel disappointment or any other emotion. And their response is 100 percent based on their conditioning, their life experiences up until now, just as yours is. You have never walked in anyone else's shoes, nor have they walked in yours. You have no idea what it is like to be them or what emotional patterns they run. If they choose disappointment, well, they choose disappointment. It is just an emotion and it will pass. Many women feel guilty because they believe they are not a good enough friend, partner, wife, mother, daughter, sister, colleague… and it gets you nowhere. The first step to change your exhausting emotional responses, the ones that don't serve you, is awareness. And although you may still throw to guilt, you can catch yourself. You can recognize much sooner that you've responded to a situation with guilt and rather than letting it linger and permeate your life, your relationships, and your self-esteem, you can realise you have simply told yourself your old story. Make this one of your mental go-to statements… only if I were to indulge in the debilitating, exhausting, health-depleting emotion of guilt will I feel it, instead of remembering that I haven't walked in anyone else's shoes, cannot control how they will respond to my words or actions, and that only I determine how I feel.

From this point on, begin to become aware of the stories you tell yourself. They are simply that, stories. And remember you have zero control over how someone reacts to what you do or say. Guilt is exhausting. Become aware of how often you feel it. Notice if guilt motivates you or makes you want to stay at home and eat. Or if you attempt to distract yourself from the guilt you feel through your nightly few glasses of wine. Start to notice…

A rushing woman needs to spend far more time with her PNS activated. How can she do this? For a start, she has to get real about how much caffeine she drinks. Many women warm up with caffeine and cool down with alcohol. Women are exhausted on waking and need help relaxing in the evening. Vicious cycle isn't it?

HOW DO WOMEN BECOME SNS DOMINANT?

There are numerous roads to an SNS dominant life, and some of them involve a high or low level of a particular physical substance, such as caffeine or progesterone, while others are the result of our emotional landscape and the behaviours we display which are 100 percent due to our beliefs. Trouble is, most of us are totally unconscious to what we really believe. Later chapters will offer assistance with the emotional side of things while below is a summary of the physical aspects of our lifestyles that can lead to SNS dominance.

Caffeine

I wish it weren't so, believe me! But yes, caffeine is the fastest and surest way to amp up that SNS response. And how many people start their day with a caffeinated beverage? More than 90 percent of people in the Western world consume caffeine every day. It is a powerful nervous system drug and it also drives the adrenal glands to produce adrenalin, the hormone that promotes the sympathetic nervous system to stay in the red alert alarm state. Caffeine demands your body use glucose as its fuel, drawing on glucose in the blood or drawing the stored version of glucose (glycogen) out of the liver and the muscles into the blood to be used as the fuel in this highly alert state.

What I've observed in so many women is that if their day is calm, non-chaotic and without pressure or demands, and caffeine is thrown into that mix, then the caffeine still stimulates (as that is its mechanism of action), but not to the point of overwhelm… and overwhelm can show up as snappy, impatient behaviour or sadness and withdrawal. But how do you know when a day may present with challenges and therefore if it might be "safer" to have a caffeinated drink? One client described it beautifully…

> *I like to start my day with a latte that I make myself. I sometimes then buy a coffee mid-morning when I'm out and about. If I*

don't speak to anyone all day, I feel OK. I do notice my energy crashes about two hours after the second coffee but as far as the feelings of overwhelm go, they don't kick in. But these days, at the age of forty-one, I only have to get a phone call from my husband, and if he is panicked about something or seems frustrated with me, I can't stop shaking on the inside after I hang up. I feel like the smallest task on my to-do list is overwhelming and I make mountains out of molehills for the rest of the day. I even end up in tears feeling like I can't cope when I felt fine when I woke up. When I came to see you about my periods, you asked me to take a break from coffee for two menstrual cycles. Not only did my pre-menstrual tension (PMT) go away but those feelings, even when my husband was worked up, did not arise the whole time I was off coffee. I can't tell you the difference it has made to my day and to my health. I now have one coffee on the weekend if my husband and I take the children out for breakfast but it took that break for me to realise that the coffee was like the straw that broke this camel's back!

Step one to taking the load off your SNS is to take

a break from coffee and, at first, switch to green tea. It does contain caffeine (about 30mg) but much less than coffee (about 80mg in an espresso-based drink), plus it is rich in anti-oxidants, has significant anti-cancer properties, and benefits the liver. Some rushing women find that even green tea is too stimulating, so once you have weaned off coffee using green tea, you can switch to herbal teas that contain no caffeine if you need to. Or simply make warm water with lemon as your hot drink.

Low Progesterone

When a woman's sex hormones are out of balance, it can feel to her like the world will end. She can feel "out of her body," as if she has no grounding and like there's something wrong but she doesn't know what it is. Progesterone clearly has a reproductive role to play in our body, however, it plays many other roles as well. In our body, progesterone behaves like an antidepressant and an antianxiety agent, and it is crucial for clear thinking. In the fourteen years I have worked with people one-on-one about their health and nutrition, I have seen six women with optimal progesterone levels. Six! In fourteen years! I know I see a biased group of the population... no one comes to see a health professional like me when they feel fabulous and everything in their world is perfect. All

I want to say is that it has become common but not normal for a woman's progesterone to be low and that can mean any or all of the following: low mood, unexplained weight gain, an inability to lose weight despite excellent food and movement patterns, challenges conceiving, fluid retention, poor thyroid function, or an anxious feeling inside her body that she can't explain. And if she stops to think about it, she can't work out if the feeling like she never gets it all done and can never quite manage to keep everyone happy that she wishes she could... she can't work out if the anxious feeling came first or if something is causing that. And from a scientific perspective it can be either. It can be that all of the rushing brought on the anxious feeling, as year after year living your life as a rushing woman is a surefire way to deplete your progesterone levels. My point is, however, that low progesterone levels can also lead us to rush as progesterone physically helps to keep women calm. It is a classic chicken or egg situation.

Lack of Sleep

There are a few things I link to amazing health. Optimal nutrition, of course, fresh air, movement, love, forgiveness, and great sleep. Sleep affects our physical and mental health. One link that is particularly relevant to many of us is that between good quality sleep and stress management. Sleep is often the only time our bodies are able to access the rest and repair part of our nervous system (the PNS). Sleep is critical for skin regeneration, immunity, hair growth, nail growth, and all other non-vital processes the body will not prioritize during the day, particularly when under constant stress and SNS activation. For many of us when we put our head on the pillow at night, it may be the first time that day we feel we have truly stopped. Yet the more tasks that pile up on our to-do list, the more we tend to sacrifice the one thing that allows our PNS to become dominant again... sleep. When I would run programs at health retreats, I would often ask people what they loved most about their week. One of the most common answers I received was "sleep." Going to bed at a good time and getting up at the same time each morning, usually with the sun, sends a powerful message to your endocrine system, the system that involves all of the glands that regulate your incredibly important bodily functions like reproduction and the stress response. When you don't sleep enough, you don't allow your PNS to have as much of a chance to be the dominant arm of the nervous system. So for people who live their lives with an urgency, a hurriedness that their friends and colleagues may or may not witness (many women hide the panic away inside), the time they are asleep may be the only time they give their PNS the opportunity to drive the ship.

Yet for many SNS dominant women, they can't sleep properly or they do not feel sleep restores them. Remember that when you are in an SNS-dominant state, your body tends to churn out stress hormones and if one of those stress hormones is screaming to every cell of your body that your life is in danger, which is what adrenalin does, your body will never let you sleep deeply because it wants you to survive the imminent attack it perceives. So it is a vicious cycle. Sleep is difficult to restore to excellent quality if you don't first allow the PNS to become the dominant arm of the nervous system. Reestablishing restorative sleep is a major benefit that comes from addressing Rushing Woman's Syndrome.

Over-Exercising

As mentioned earlier, certain types of exercise can seem like more stress to an already over-stressed human body. Do you think our ancestors woke up and thought it would be a great day for a run? No! Running meant we were attempting to escape from danger back then, while now it has become a way to burn off the excesses a Western lifestyle "affords" us. I'm not saying running is bad, for those of you who love it. Barefoot running, in particular, certainly promotes being present in the moment and there is certainly a science that can be applied to running to promote fat burning and nervous system calm. I'm simply saying that if running and high-intensity exercise (combined with good eating) hasn't shifted your weight by now, it is not suddenly going to start doing so until some other work on your body's chemistry and nervous system is done.

Even though you know you are just exercising intensely, from your body's perspective, once the threat (perceived by your body to be present due to the release of stress hormones) is dealt with, the PNS slows our heart rate and respiration back down, brings the blood back to the digestive tract so that we can digest our food, works to repair any tissue damage, and increases libido. Night time is when the parasympathetic system has lots of time to do its job, provided we go to bed early enough. As you have read earlier, the sympathetic and parasympathetic systems are supposed to balance each other nicely, and in those people who have a balanced nervous system, high-intensity exercise will lead to fat loss, as the parasympathetic rest time between workouts is when muscle tissue is built.

Those who are unable to lose fat by doing regular high-intensity exercise may have a dominant sympathetic nervous system, and, consequently, an inhibited parasympathetic system. There is too much systemic stress coming from somewhere, and for those people adding high-intensity exercise is counterproductive, as it adds to their sympathetic load, pushing them even more out of balance. Instead you want to decrease the sympathetic load by reducing stressors and choosing an exercise that is done slowly and with the breath, such as restorative yoga, qi gong, tai chi, yoga, feldenkrais or Alexander technique. These activities will increase the parasympathetic system and help balance the ANS. The goal is to balance the nervous system so that when you do need to rush, you can, but then leave the rush, and all its health-depleting effects, behind.

Lack of Solitude

Another factor that can lead to SNS dominance is a lack of solitude, time spent on your own. When I talk about being alone I don't mean feeling lonely. They are different things. In fact, science has demonstrated some of the health benefits that come from spending time in solitude. It decreases stress hormones and has been shown to boost memory, creativity, mood, and empathy. It allows us to recharge. On the inside this means that the PNS gets to have its time in the sun being dominant, where the vital rest, repair, and digest processes can do their work. When we rest and repair the body is able to choose between sugar and fat as its fuel, and it usually chooses both. That is a good thing. Health problems can occur when the body feels as if it has no choice but to always choose glucose for its fuel.

How can you seek solitude in your day? Going for a walk by yourself and noticing the nature around you is a great place to start. If you live with other people and you have the house to yourself, even if it is only once a week for a brief period of time, allow yourself to stop for at least some of that time, even though you will feel like "making the most of it to get more jobs done." You may feel that I cannot possibly understand your life and how busy you are. But part of what I want to show you is that when you create a spaciousness in your life, you *feel* like you have more time, and you no longer have to rush.

It may not feel possible for you right now, particularly if you have small children. Often when they rest you need to rest, too, although so many women rush around even more while their baby sleeps, to get on top of the jobs that have piled up! One way to look at it is to give yourself permission to rest on two out of the seven days of the week, while your baby sleeps. For the other five, you can choose to do tasks or to rest. Or you may prefer to start with one day of rest and increase this by one day every second week, until you have three rest days a week. Small steps can feel much more manageable. Another important thing to consider is that children are little for such a relatively short time. If you feel like right now you just can't take some time in solitude, you will soon be able to. If you feel like this then perhaps while they sleep, you can at least sit for five minutes and focus on your breathing. More begets more remember? It can be practical to start small with your solitude if you feel like it is a far-off dream.

Excess Liver Loaders

In my book *Accidentally Overweight* one of the nine factors I linked to using body fat as a fuel was optimal liver function. "Stress" on the physical body can also play a role in pushing us into SNS dominance through a variety of scientific mechanisms, the details of which I explained in *Accidentally Overweight*. But rather than focusing on the mechanisms here, I simply want you to know that some foods and certain beverages can promote a stress response inside us. For example, you may notice your heart races after you've had too much wine in one sitting for your body to detoxify. Countless women tell me that they notice their heart racing once they go to bed after they have had alcohol. The main liver loaders are listed below. They include:

- Alcohol
- Caffeine
- Trans fats
- Sugars, including fructose and sucrose
- Synthetic substances, such as pesticides, medications, skin "care"
- Infection, for example viruses such as glandular fever (Epstein-Barr virus, Mononucleosis)

Some of these you have a choice about, some not so. When it comes to the amount of alcohol, caffeine and refined sugars in your diet, you know when you are having too much... and I mean too much for you. The amount tolerated by one person is likely to be different from another and you know better than anyone when you are having too much of anything. Even as you read this, if something has welled up inside you, your body's wisdom is letting you know. Knowledge is one thing; action is another thing entirely. Taking action to lower or omit your liver loaders for a period of time can make a significant difference to the rush and its health consequences. More on this later...

Alcohol is a big issue for many rushing women.

Many are exhausted, overwhelmed, and haven't had any time to themselves for at least five or twenty-five years, that alcohol is, to paraphrase many of my clients, "my only pleasure in the day," "the only way I can relax at the end of the day," "something for me... the only thing just for me in my day," "the only way I get any peace," "reward for all of my efforts over the day." I ask women who drink every night to finish the sentence, "Alcohol is..." and those are some of the things they say. Reality is alcohol is none of those things. They are meanings *you* have given alcohol. These are the stories you tell yourself about why you need it, why it is OK to have it every night of your life. I don't believe the female body in particular was ever designed to consume alcohol most nights of its adult life. And women are experiencing the consequences of the regular, overconsumption of it, with this type of drinking now highly associated with five of our biggest cancers. The links are undeniable. But for many of you, even scientific fact that the regular, overconsumption of alcohol (amounts outlined later) significantly increases your risk of breast cancer won't stop you from telling yourself that it is your "only pleasure in the day." Ladies, seriously. If the only thing you derive pleasure from in your entire day is an alcoholic drink, it is time for a new perspective. As an aside, many women repeat the same statements to me about coffee or a particular type of food. This is not about taking away your fun or your pleasure. I simply want you to be able to choose how much and how often you you consume these liver loaders, rather than your desire for them being ruled by your emotional state… for then you feel out of control of often regret your food or drink choices.

CHOICE

We have so much to be thankful for. I encourage you to be truly thankful *every* day for the privilege of living in a peaceful country. Every night before you go to sleep, take a moment to simply be grateful for what you *do* have and not worry about what you may not have. Take some time out *every* day to have an "attitude of gratitude." We are so blessed to live in a society where we have an amazing array of choices available each day… more than our ancestors would ever have dreamed possible. And, it is likely that anyone reading this, no matter how they may perceive their own life at present, still has a lifestyle that millions in the world would wish could be theirs. Many people don't have fresh water to drink. It's also easy to take choice for granted particularly when life doesn't work out quite the way we had planned. We have opportunities to shape our futures but we don't always have control over unexpected events. We would never consciously choose for ourselves or those we love to have an accident, a serious illness, job loss, or to be involved in a natural disaster. But, even if challenges present themselves, we must never forget that we retain control over our attitude toward that event. When I talk with people about their perception of choice, I am fascinated, occasionally saddened, but mostly inspired by the immense power of the human spirit. Here is one such response . . .

> *When my parents died when I was sixteen, I had no choice in the circumstance. However, I was faced with other choices... to seek the so-called comfort of drugs or the true support of friends, to be negative or positive, to look backward or forward. Although I had absolutely no choice surrounding the situation I found myself in, I still had a choice in terms of what attitude I adopted. I knew that whatever choice I made wouldn't bring them back so I simply chose to get on with my own life as best I could. Admittedly, there were times when I doubted I would succeed in doing so but there is no comparison between that which is lost by not succeeding and that, which is lost by not trying. With no family to fall back on, or blame, I learned earlier than*

most that I was totally responsible for my own choices for the rest of my life. Because of the volunteer work I've ended up doing in the later part of my life, I've walked the beat with police as rocks were hurled at us, been called to an armed robbery, intervened in domestic violence situations and sat for hours on a drug bust. Perpetrators of those crimes made different choices than me but I suspend judgment because I may have made the same choices once, and I give thanks that I didn't. Choices have given me more than my fair share of joy and sorrow. But even in my darkest moments, I remind myself to give thanks for that freedom to choose.

Every day, I am truly grateful for so much in my life, such as fresh air, freedom, and real food. I'm equally grateful for the things I don't have, like persecution, hunger, and disease. Every day, it is worth reminding ourselves that the choices are ours. I cannot encourage you enough to spend time each day focusing on the things for which you are grateful. Share that gratitude with others. And remember to include the things that aren't in your life for which you are grateful too. As Tony Robbins so accurately says, "what you focus on is what you feel." And if you tell yourself that alcohol is the only pleasurable thing in your entire day, then it will be, yet there is so much more on offer, around you and within you every minute of every day and night. It is just that when you are exhausted and running on the caffeine, sugar, alcohol highway of sub-optimal nutrition and SNS dominance, racing around everywhere with your to-do list never being all checked off, it can be quite a challenge to remember how magnificent your life truly is.

Yet when you allow the PNS to be dominant, whether that is through less caffeine, sorting out your sex hormone balance, going to bed earlier or scheduling some "yin" type movement in your day. Exploring and resolving elements of your emotional landscape are also going to assist. And from the spaciousness that PNS dominance promotes, you cannot only see the magnificence and the wonder, but you can feel it within, just as you did as a very little girl. Your rituals create your life. Get some good ones!

LIFE A LONG TIME AGO... AND LIFE TODAY

There is an age-old inclination wired into us to protect, hoard, and defend. The enemy is lurking, waiting to eat you, annihilate you. The part of our brain linked to the fight or flight response, known as the reptilian brain—despite being augmented by the limbic brain (a different part of the brain linked to emotions) and the neocortex (yet another part of our very clever brain)—is still focused on physical survival, the fight or flight. And when we allow our most basic impulses, the very ones that helped the earliest humans survive, to direct the higher brain centres, we act like lizards. And given we were born with the inclination to do whatever is needed to survive, we need to respect the genius of a brain that has done its job and brought us this far. But we also need to update our wiring since the chances of being eaten by a lion are slim, even though when we rush, our body's perception is that that big cat is actually very real! Being on red alert has now become maladaptive because it causes us to live in a constant state of tension, which is unhealthy and therefore counterproductive to our survival. Only our nervous system, of which our brain is a part, hasn't been able to keep up with the rate of change or the pace of life the Western world now asks of us. So for now, until our evolution can catch up (can it ever?), we have to choose to support the part of our nervous system that dissolves tension as long as we make it feel like it is safe to do so.

There is a wonderful analogy I love to use to describe how people have become oblivious to the stress and pressure in their lives. It is about a frog and as green tree frogs just happen to be one of my favourite creatures on the planet (and one of my nicknames is Frog), it appeals to me even more! The analogy is this, origin unknown but thought to be based on a scientific experiment published in 1897…

If you put a frog in cool water it swims around very happily. If you put a frog in boiling water it immediately jumps out to save itself. But if you put a frog in cool water and slowly bring that water to the boil, the frog doesn't notice and doesn't jump out.

I believe that most people in the Western world would jump out of the pressure in their lives if they were suddenly thrown into it. But we don't jump out when it gradually increases over the years. We don't tend to notice until a crisis hits… the death of someone we love or our own health crashes. Don't let it take a health crisis to wake you up to the fact that without your health you have nothing. If you recognize that you are like a frog whose world has been on the boil, act now to change it. Begin to put strategies in place to change either your situation or your perception of your life, or both. This book will cover many options open to you. Either way, the changes it will foster in your biochemistry, your emotional landscape, and hence your health, are potentially enormous.

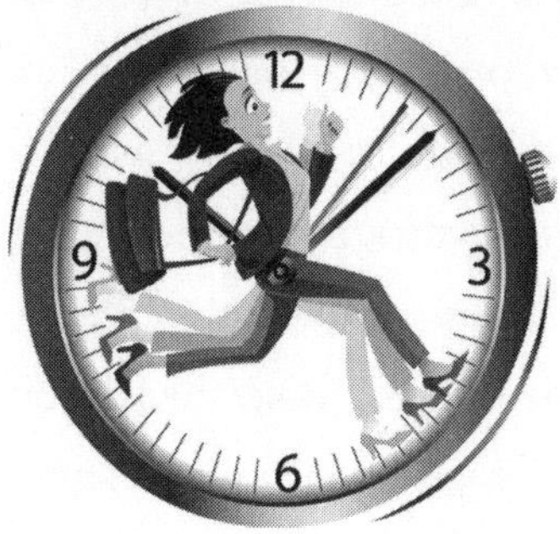

Chapter 3
The Endocrine System

This is a little bit of science made simple to help you on your way with this chapter. This section needs a little bit of setup before we get into the juicy bits that lead to the ah-ha moments that will help you understand what might be going on in your body.

THE ENDOCRINE GLANDS

The endocrine system is made up of numerous glands that secrete hormones, including the pituitary, thyroid, parathyroids, adrenals, and the reproductive organs; the ovaries in women and the testes in men, although the latter two are technically not endocrine glands exclusively. But for the purpose of explaining the role of the endocrine system in rushing, they will be included as they play a vital role in how we feel and function on a daily basis.

Around the age of twelve, as they enter puberty, boys and girls start to develop striking differences in physical appearance and behaviour. Perhaps no other period in life so clearly demonstrates the impact of both the nervous system and the endocrine system in directing development and regulating body functions. Changes in the brain and pituitary gland markedly increase the synthesis of new messenger molecules, the sex hormones, from the gonads. In girls, fatty tissue starts to accumulate in the breasts and hips. At the same time, or a little later, in boys, protein synthesis increases, muscle mass builds, and the longer, larger vocal cords start producing a lower-pitched voice. These changes provide just a few examples of the powerful influence of the secretions from endocrine glands.

THE CO-ORDINATION OF THE NERVOUS AND ENDOCRINE SYSTEMS

Together, the nervous and endocrine systems coordinate functions of all body systems. The nervous system controls homeostasis (the point where all things are in balance) through nerve impulses, while the endocrine system releases its messenger molecules (called hormones) into the bloodstream.

The circulating blood then delivers hormones to virtually all cells throughout the body. The nervous and endocrine systems are coordinated as an interlocking super system, referred to as the neuroendocrine system. Certain parts of the nervous system stimulate or inhibit the release of hormones from the glands of the endocrine system. Hormones may then, in turn, promote or inhibit the generation of nerve impulses. Also, several molecules act as hormones in some locations and as neurotransmitters in others.

The nervous system causes muscles to contract and glands to secrete more or less of their products. The endocrine system alters metabolic activities, regulates growth and development, and guides reproductive processes. It therefore not only helps regulate the activity of things like smooth and cardiac muscle and some glands, it significantly affects virtually all other tissues in the body as well.

Nerve impulses tend to produce their effects within a few milliseconds. While some hormones can act within seconds, others can take up to several hours or more to bring about their responses. Also, the effects of stimulating the nervous system are generally brief compared with those of the endocrine system. So with that out of the way, let's get into the details of how the endocrine system affects you; how you look, feel, and function every day.

Firstly I want you to know that the pituitary gland, housed inside a part of your brain, is the master gland, or the switch of the endocrine system. Technically, the hypothalamus, an organ with some endocrine tissue within it, influences the function of the pituitary, however, for ease of explanation and to keep the Rushing Woman's Syndrome message concise, the hypothalamus won't be explored in detail. It is briefly discussed in the pituitary section within the endocrine chapter.

The pituitary gland sends the signals out to your other endocrine system glands, alerting them to the hormones they need to make. Likewise, the thyroid talks to the ovaries. The adrenals and the ovaries also have a relationship and on and on the chatter inside you goes. That's what hormones do... they talk... they send messages, and each of those messages communicates information to the different cells, tissues, and organs inside your body. Nothing, and I mean nothing, works alone. Everything is influenced by something else.

So the importance of the coming sections—about the adrenal glands and the stress hormones they make, the ovaries and the sex hormones they make, the thyroid gland and the temperature-controlling, metabolism-influencing hormones it makes, as well as the master of them all, the pituitary—is enormous and will open your mind and your heart to a whole new way to view your health and the pace of our lives as well as provide you with insights and support to make the changes you feel inspired to make. Hormonal systems… here we come!

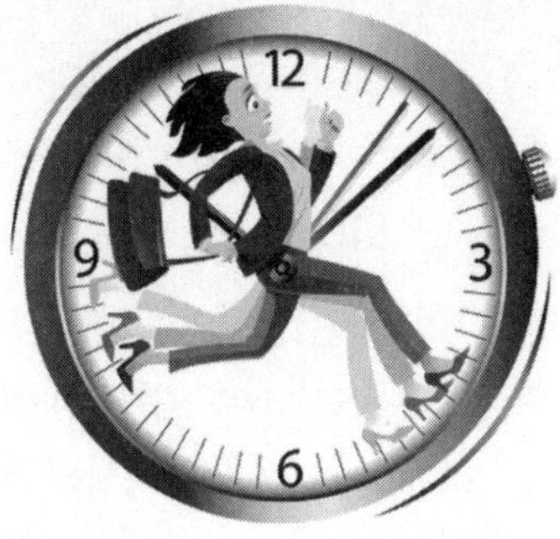

Chapter 3 Part 1

Your Adrenal Glands and Your Stress Hormones: their role and impact on you in your rush

When you tell me that you delete emails off your phone while sitting on the toilet because that's good time management, I can tell you, with love and respect, that you are a rushing woman. When I first started to work with people on their health, consultations were comparatively calm. Fourteen years ago, women would arrive (mostly) on time, relatively unhurried, and, if they had a cell phone, they turned it off. Now, they rush in, (mostly) have impatience and urgency pouring out in their energy until at least fifteen minutes into the consultation, their cell phones ring and ping with calls and emails, and if I could make a sound that described them, it would be a high-pitched whizzing whir. Yes, I'm generalizing and of course some women put their phones on silent for our session. However, I'm describing a general trend to make a point. Women are stretched and stressed and time poor like never before. Yes, we can argue that there has always been stress. But it has never before come in the constant, urgent avalanche that has become the norm for so many women in the Western world. So let's look at what we ask of our body from an adrenal and stress hormone perspective when we live in this way. For those of you who read my book *Accidentally Overweight*, some of this information was covered there but this section has been expanded and is essential reading at this stage in the Rushing Woman's journey so you can appreciate the powerful role your adrenal glands play in your health, body shape and size, your vitality, and your sense of calm and coping.

Your adrenal glands are two very precious, walnut-sized glands that sit just on top of your kidneys. They may be small in stature, but the power they pack when they are working optimally is an energetic, health gift to us all. The adrenal glands produce many hormones, two of which are your stress hormones, namely adrenaline (known as epinephrine in the USA) and cortisol.

ADRENALIN, THE RUSH, AND THE BIG SUGAR RUSH

Adrenalin is your short-term, acute stress hormone. It is the one that's produced when you get a fright. If someone suddenly runs into the room and startles you and you jump, that feeling that most of us know very well is caused by adrenalin. Adrenalin is designed to get you out of danger—and get you out of danger fast. Historically, we made adrenalin when our life was being threatened, and our response, fuelled by adrenalin, was typically physical. A tiger might have suddenly jumped out of the jungle at you or perhaps a member of another tribe started chasing you with a spear. In that moment, you made adrenalin to get out of danger. Adrenalin promotes what is known as the "fight or flight" response. When activated, the typically excellent blood supply to your digestive system is diverted away from your digestive system to your periphery, to your arms and your legs. This is necessary because you need a powerful blood supply to your arms and legs to get you out of danger. You also need fuel to give them the necessary energy; the most readily available fuel is glucose, often referred to as sugar (a carbohydrate). Your liver and your muscles store glucose in the form of glycogen, and adrenalin communicates to your liver and your muscles that energy is required. They then convert glycogen back into glucose and dump this glucose into your blood. Your blood sugar subsequently shoots up, ready to fuel your self-defence or your escape. And you feel amped.

This cascade of events—and the biochemical changes that result—allows you to escape from danger in a very active way. Regardless of the outcome, regardless of whether you win that challenge or not (you escape, die, or win the fight), this stress, the threat to your life, and the need for adrenalin is over very quickly. The trouble is that for many of us in the modern world, it is more often psychological stress that drives us to make adrenalin. And so although our life may not literally be threatened, this hormone still communicates to every cell of our body that our life is indeed at risk. Adrenalin makes your heart race, your thoughts race, and gives you a jittery feeling that can make it difficult to feel calm despite your best efforts.

Psychological stress can come in many forms. It may be that you return from a week away from work to find seven hundred new emails in your in-box, and you wonder when on earth you're going to find the time to deal with those. It may be that your landline rings and, while you take that call, your mobile rings, and you feel that you can barely finish one conversation before demands begin to start another. If you are sitting in front of your computer while all of this is going on, and a few emails also arrive in your in-box while you juggle the incoming demands and noise, the adrenaline tends to climb higher. Perhaps you set your alarm for the morning, you press snooze… you keep pressing snooze and suddenly you sit bolt upright in bed and realize you're running late. You may still have to iron clothes, prepare lunches, deliver little people to school and, because you're leaving later than usual, you get stuck in traffic. Meanwhile, your mobile phone starts ringing with people at the office wondering where you are as you are supposed to be in a meeting, but you are stuck in the middle of rush hour traffic, and your brain has gone into overdrive with the enormity of your morning. And you've only been up for an hour!

When you finally burst through the doors at work, all you can think about is how much you want a coffee. So all morning you've been making adrenalin, and now you are going to make even more adrenalin, as caffeine promotes its production. All you actually want from the "coffee" at this point in your day is a little breathing space, a moment in time just for you. The reasons we crave a hot drink may vary, but often it's just to catch our breath. In those coffee break moments, it is as if there is a bubble around us, and we are silently communicating, "Don't you dare come near me for the next three minutes!" I've had countless women tell me that coffee is the only peace they get in their day, which if you look at the reality of it, is not true, as physically coffee is adding to the demand on your adrenal glands to produce adrenalin to get you out of danger that doesn't actually exist.

One important difference between the past and modern day is that the biochemical changes generated by adrenalin, such as sugar being dumped into your blood to get you out of danger, serve a useful purpose while you are physically fighting or fleeing. If you're sitting on your bottom at your desk in front of a computer and sugar is being dumped into your blood, you make insulin to deal with that elevation in blood sugar. And insulin is one of our primary fat storage hormones. Not only that but it sets your blood sugar up to crash at a later stage, creating a fatigued state that makes you feel like only more caffeine or high sugar food can fix. You can see that adrenalin is a significant hormone that sets us up to keep rushing.

HOW COFFEE AMPS YOU UP

Over 90 percent of adults in the Western world consume caffeine daily. More than 50 percent of Americans consume thirteen or more caffeinated drinks per week. In Australia and New Zealand studies suggest caffeine consumption has more than tripled since the 1960s and although levels may not be on par with rates of consumption in the U.S., they are rapidly rising due to an increase in coffee consumption plus the widespread use of caffeine as an ingredient in, for example, energy drinks. In the U.S., 70 percent of soft drinks contain caffeine. In a U.S. study conducted in 2011, 28 percent of coffee drinkers had their first cup within 15 minutes of waking and 68 percent within an hour of waking, while 57 percent added sugar or sweetener to their brew. The level of caffeine consumption for far too many people is considered to be "addictive" by medical standards.

When you consume caffeine, it sends a message to the pituitary gland in your brain that it needs to send a message to the adrenal glands to make adrenalin. When adrenalin is released, your blood sugar elevates to provide you with more energy, your blood pressure and pulse rate rise to provide more oxygen to the muscles, which tense in preparation for action. Reproductive functions are downregulated since they use a lot of energy and are not necessary for your immediate survival, given the impending threat. Plus, your body does not believe it is "safe" to bring a baby into what your body perceives is an unsafe world. Not when your stress hormones are telling your body that your life is in danger (adrenalin) or that there is no more food left in the world (cortisol, which will be explained on a moment)!

Adrenalin production can be the result of real or perceived stress, or simply the result of your caffeine intake. Caffeine, via stress hormones and coupled with the signal to activate your sympathetic nervous system (remembering sugar fuels this arm of the nervous system) fires you up. Once triggered, you have little hope of being calm, centred, and able to focus on instructions being given to you (e.g. by your boss, or a colleague, or a receptionist confirming an appointment with you) in this state. In addition, this biochemical state can either lead you to slenderness or fat storage, because insulin—the fat storage hormone—will firstly convert unused glucose from your blood into glycogen and store it in your muscles and what is left over will be converted into body fat. Let me explain this with the story of a client I'll call Susan.

This strikingly slim and physically beautiful woman had an appointment to see me. I did what I do with every client and asked how I could help her and what she would like to get out of our session. Susan apologized for what she thought would sound vain and said that she had gained three kilos (seven pounds) recently and was seeing me because nothing in her diet or activity level had changed and could be attributed to the weight gain. She was concerned that she may be perimenopausal even though her periods had not changed. She said some of her friends had gained weight during perimenopause and she was here because she was concerned that those three kilos would become ten before she knew it, if she didn't get to the bottom of why her body had changed. I admired Susan's attitude and her desire to understand her body better. We discussed the many facets of her life, emotional and physical, and when it came time to talk about her food, her diet was outstanding with regards to all of my benchmarks for eating a diet based on fresh foods. People like me have numerous strategies that we can apply to assist someone in their quest for fat loss; from a food perspective this lady was already living by most of the tricks of my trade. When it came time to talk about her liquid intake, she politely informed me that she had one glass of red wine four times per week and that she had done this with her husband for years. And then I asked if she drank coffee. Susan's eyes lit up. She replied that, yes, she loved it, but acknowledged, on reflection, that her caffeine intake *was* something that had changed. She had always had a coffee before breakfast every day for most of her adult life, and that was the only caffeine she consumed all day. But for the past three to four months, she had begun to have up to four coffees per day, but she didn't know why. She just had. When my eyes lit up back at her, she quickly justified her intake by saying, "But they are all black coffees, so there are no calories in them." She drank them all at her desk. She had never exercised, and I could see that she had very little muscle mass. Her fat had gone on around her tummy.

Susan could see from the look on my face where I was about to go and, before I'd even spoken, she said "Please don't take them from me." I wanted her to see how emotionally attached she was so I didn't interrupt her. Eventually, I said that I believed it was the coffee that had led to the change in her body, and she cried. She literally cried. She told me it was impossible, and she kept coming back to the calorie reasoning. She basically had a tantrum in my office. I gently tried to lead her to the truth that actually it's only a drink, yet she behaved as if her four daily coffees held the meaning of life for her. I then went on to explain the mechanism I outlined above involving caffeine, adrenalin, elevated blood sugar, and subsequent insulin production. I told her that I wasn't even asking her to give up caffeine entirely. My clients will tell you that, when it is warranted, I often ask them to give up caffeine completely for a four-week trial period. They are often shocked by how much more energy they have without caffeine in their lives. I simply wanted this client to go back to her one cup a day before breakfast, a coffee prepared with love by her husband, to see what happened. Susan agreed to make this change for four weeks, even though she couldn't imagine anything being more powerful than calories in fat creation and couldn't see how this plan could possibly work. I did nothing else for this woman. Not one other change to her dietary intake and, four weeks later, she burst through my door telling me she had lost four kilos (nine pounds) in four weeks. She had only gained three (seven pounds) in the first place. As an aside, I have never weighed a client nor will I ever weigh a client as I believe you simply weigh your self-esteem when you do.

My theory was that Susan's weight gain was the result of the perception of her nervous system, rather than the result of too many calories. Her subsequent weight loss was, in my opinion, extremely fast, but my point in sharing this story with you is to demonstrate caffeine's power to signal what is, for some, fat storage and an almost crazed emotional state, of which her tantrum when we first met was demonstrative. Decreasing her coffee consumption seemed like an overwhelming task for her. Granted, the fast weight loss will not happen for everyone but the level of calm certainly improves with less caffeine. Weight loss is significantly dependent on the balance between your sympathetic and your parasympathetic nervous systems.

It is so important that you consider your caffeine habits and get honest with yourself about how it affects you. Does it dull your appetite and so unconsciously you grab a coffee instead of eating? This is especially true for many women at lunchtime. Does it make your heart race, give you the shakes, or loosen your bowels? Does it elevate your blood pressure? Do you notice you want it more when you are stressed and, if so, what story have you attached to what coffee gives you? Do you have restless, poor quality sleep because of how much caffeine you consume? Or does it lift your mood or nourish your soul with no ill effect whatsoever? You know yourself better than anyone. Act on what you know is true for you.

Think about all of these mechanisms. So many of us run on adrenalin. Moment to moment, day to day, it's like a light switch has gone on, and it hasn't entirely switched off for a really long time. And it doesn't have to be traumatic stress and shocking situations that drive this process in us. It can simply be the pace at which we live our lives; the juggling act that leads so many women I meet to say that they want more "balance" in their lives, that they can't cope like this anymore and that their perception is that their "stress is killing them."

The human body is incredibly resilient and although we were not designed to withstand long-term stress (due to the way we're designed, we are healthier when it is short-lived), many bodies appear to tolerate, as opposed to thrive on, years and years of living on adrenalin. Yet I have witnessed firsthand what the relentless production of this hormone is doing to women's health, including impacting their fertility, PMS and the severity of it, their digestive systems, and their relationships. An additional challenge, however, is that once the body perceives that the stress has become long-term, your dominant stress hormone begins to change.

CORTISOL—FRIEND OR WORST NIGHTMARE

Cortisol is your long-term stress hormone. Historically, the only long-term stress humans had revolved around food being scarce. Long-term stress came in the form of floods, famines, and wars. During such times, a person didn't know where the next meal was coming from. Today, in the Western world, our long-term stresses tend to be more along the lines of financial pressure or relationship concerns, and uncertainty or worries about our health—even our weight. For so many women, their first waking thoughts involve "What will I or won't I eat today?" or "How much exercise can I get done today?"

Or, for some, the thoughts might speed along like this: "Oh, my goodness, it's Wednesday, and I still haven't been to the gym, and, my gosh, it's 7:00pm and there's no food at home, which means I still have to go to the supermarket, and if I go to the supermarket that means I won't get home until 8:30pm and then I have to cook and clean up and then it will be midnight before I get to bed and I have to get up at a good time to get to work early in the morning, but I'm going to a party in three weeks and I really wanted to fit into my favourite red dress and that's not going to happen because I haven't been to the gym all week and I am still not going to go tonight because otherwise I won't get any sleep and get to work on time to do everything I have to do..." and on and on and on it goes. So many women live like this most days of their life. When it happens day after day it can easily lead to a chronic pattern of stress response, hence increased cortisol output, which in turn can lead to a change in your metabolism and essentially your behaviour, because not only do you feel like you can't keep up but your body's perception is that it has to do everything at a rapid pace.

It is important to understand how cortisol works, as it can be your friend or one of your worst nightmares. When made at optimum amounts, cortisol does numerous wonderful things for your health. It is one of the body's primary anti-inflammatory mediators, meaning that wherever there is inflammation in the body, cortisol, having been converted into cortisone, dampens down the effect of that inflammation and stops your body from feeling stiff, rigid, or in pain. Many people, for example, will describe the feeling that they have suddenly aged as they come out of difficult times, often the result of sub-optimal cortisol levels during such periods. In the right amount, cortisol is not only an anti-inflammatory, it also buffers the effect of insulin, meaning that optimum amounts help you continue to burn body fat for energy while also maintaining stable—as opposed to rapidly fluctuating—blood sugar levels.

Cortisol levels change over the day. The right amount assists you with various bodily functions throughout the course of the day. Cortisol is designed to be high in the morning and, for the purpose of this discussion, let's say that 25 units at around 6:00am are ideal. Cortisol is one of the mechanisms that wakes you up in the morning and helps you bounce out of bed full of energy and vitality. By midday, optimum cortisol will sit at around 15 units, and, by 6:00pm, levels will ideally be at around 4 units. By 10:00pm in the evening, optimum cortisol levels are around 2 units, a level at which they are designed to stay until around 2:00am when they slowly and very steadily begin to rise again.

The following graph illustrates this. It is true what your mother told you, that one hour of sleep before midnight is worth two after, because cortisol starts to rise around 2:00am and the waking-up process gradually begins.

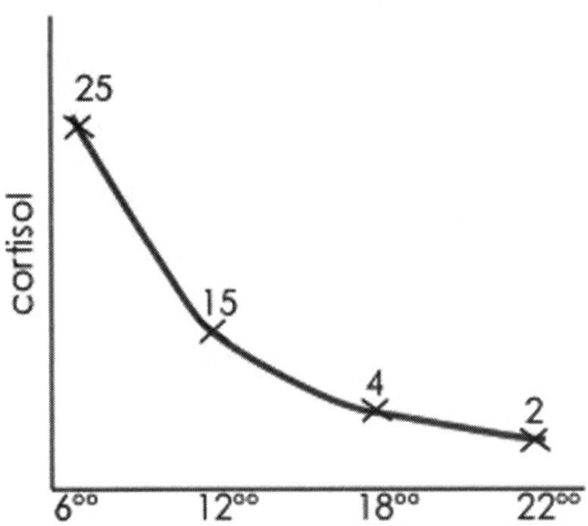

The Optimal Cortisol Profile: *Cortisol is nice and high in the morning and falls away again by the evening.*

As a stress response continues, the effect on the body begins to change. In the early stages of stress, one of the first challenges cortisol presents is that the evening level of the hormone starts to spike again rather than continue to decrease. At this stage, you still make optimum levels in the morning and are able to bounce out of bed and get on with your day with reasonable energy, but evening levels are creeping up. This is one mechanism through which good sleeping patterns can be interrupted.

When cortisol levels become elevated above optimal, other changes in body chemistry begin to unfold. It has been suggested that elevated cortisol is the one common thread behind what we have come to describe as metabolic syndrome; that is elevated blood pressure, elevated cholesterol, and insulin resistance, the latter condition (insulin) being a warning sign that if nothing changes in the near future, Type 2 diabetes is a likely consequence. If we remember that we are completely geared for survival and that cortisol tells every cell of your body that food is scarce, another of its roles is to slow down your metabolic rate. A slower metabolism leads you to burn body fat for energy far more slowly than you have in the past, as cortisol is designed to make sure that you survive this perceived period of famine.

Cortisol is "catabolic," meaning that it breaks

protein down into its building blocks, known as amino acids. This catabolism is one of the mechanisms through which cortisol slows your metabolism. Your muscles are made from proteins, and cortisol signals them to break down, as the body's perception is that fuel is needed. Additional amino acids are also needed in the blood to help repair tissues (even though you may be simply sitting on your bottom in front of the television, with your financial or relationship concerns milling around in your head!). The amino acids released as a result of the catabolic signalling of cortisol can be converted, through a process called "gluconeogenesis," back into glucose (sugar), which your body thinks may be useful to assist you in your stress. Yet if you're not active, this increase in blood glucose will not be utilized, and insulin will have to be secreted to return blood glucose levels to normal by returning the glucose in the blood to storage. Remember that glucose is stored as glycogen in the muscles and the liver.

But over time, the catabolic signalling of cortisol itself may have broken some of your muscles down, so now there is less space for glucose storage. As a result, some of the blood glucose returns to the remaining muscles while the leftovers are converted into body fat. Keeping the glucose level of the blood within the normal, safe range is of more importance to your body than whether you have wobbly bits around your middle! Essentially, too much cortisol can make you fat through dysregulated blood sugar metabolism, not just fat metabolism itself. This is one of the mechanisms through which cellulite can appear, as where muscles once were, fat can now be deposited. This is also the process through which long-term stress can lead to Type 2 diabetes.

Because cortisol is produced when the stress in your life has been going on for a while, your body (not knowing any better) thinks there is no more food left in your world, and it instinctively knows that it has a greater chance of survival if it holds on to some extra body fat. In modern times, when, for health reasons or vanity (or both), many people understand the importance of not carrying too much body fat, cortisol can provide a potential challenge to someone who believes that eating less is their only solution to body fat loss. Feeling like she is fighting an uphill battle with her body can be an immense source of stress for a woman, adding another layer of stress to her already hectic mind.

UNDERSTANDING THE CORTISOL PROBLEM

If cortisol tells every cell of your body that food is scarce, and your metabolism slows down as a result, and you continue to eat and exercise in the same way you always have, your clothes will slowly get tighter. It doesn't matter how amazingly you eat. With cortisol telling every cell in your body to store fat, it is very difficult, if not impossible, to decrease body fat until the cortisol issue is resolved. We must get to the heart of the stress and either change the situation or change the perception.

Cortisol has a very distinct fat deposition pattern. You typically lay it on around your tummy and, once again, the reason for fat placement here is governed by the body's quest for survival. If food suddenly did run out, your major organs have very easy access to fat that will keep you alive. You also tend to lay fat down on the back of the arms, and you grow what I lovingly call a back veranda. To reiterate this important point: what do most people do when they notice that their clothes are getting tighter? They go on a diet, and, when you go on a diet, do you tend to eat more or less? You typically eat less (although some audience members call out "more" when I ask them this question at a seminar!), and in doing so you reaffirm to your body that food is scarce. But food is not scarce. It is abundant for you. If you want a chocolate bar at 3:00am, you can get one. Eating less on your diet confirms to your body what it perceives to be true and that slows your metabolism even further.

Another challenge you face with elevated cortisol

coursing through your body is that, since your body thinks that food is scarce, any time you see food, it's very easy to overeat, no matter how firmly you intend to eat only three crackers when you get home from work! If that packet of crackers is open and in front of you, cortisol will scream at every cell of your body, "You are so lucky! There's food there! Eat it!" and somehow, before you know it, the whole box of crackers is gone. Please don't get me wrong… I am not saying that self-discipline and willpower have no place. My intention is simply to point out that we have very ancient hormonal mechanisms in action inside our bodies that believe they know better than you when it comes to your survival. Your body can be your biggest teacher if you learn how to decipher the messages it is communicating to you. And extra body fat is sometimes simply a vehicle of communication, just as an unjustified panicked perception of life is asking you to explore your biochemistry and your beliefs that allow this to be the case.

SILENT STRESS

What about when the stress is silent? You might not be a drama queen running around, arms flailing all over the place, screeching "I'm so stressed, I'm so stressed!" You may be a private person and keep things mostly to yourself. You may be so private with your fears and concerns, always presenting a happy face to the world, that you don't even realize that you're worried about things or recognize that you may have been in a stressed state for a very long time. You're like the boiling frog.

When you feel grateful for the life you have, it's easy to feel guilty if you complain about anything. A common internal phrase will be, "There are so many people worse off than me." This thought immediately makes you feel guilty and you stop focusing on your source of stress. Trouble is, although there *are* people worse off than you in this world, the minute you feel guilty, you change your focus so you don't ever get the opportunity to truly identify what is bothering you and, more importantly, why. These "whys" are explored in detail in the emotions section of the book. For now, I'll share a common example of keeping the peace, to help you see how everyday life, because of the perceptions we bring to it, can lead to cortisol, from an emotional source, being a contributor to your health challenges or your internal panic.

Basic psychology teaches us that humans will do more to avoid pain than they will ever do to experience pleasure. Some women I meet will do anything, for example, to keep the peace and avoid conflict. Inwardly they become highly strung because they are always walking on eggshells around others, usually their intimate partner, doing all they can to help prevent those around them from losing their temper. If the man of the house has a tendency to communicate with explosive angry outbursts that to the woman seem unpredictable, well hello silent stress hormone production! I cannot tell you how many women I've met who live like this.

Some women avoid feeling emotional pain by eating too much or making other poor food choices; perhaps by drinking bucket loads of wine or chain-smoking cigarettes. Alternatively, some people might cope or explore their pain by writing in a journal, going for a walk, a run, or a swim. Others will pray, meditate, or phone a friend and chat to deal with emotional pain. Some of the ways we cope with or explore what is going support our health. Some potentially harm our health. And all of these activities may take place with or without a conscious understanding of why.

I want to help you see *why* so that you can change your response, if it is hurting your health, especially if the stress hormone production triggered by your subconscious emotional responses is blocking either weight management or calm or both.

WORRYING IS NO GOOD FOR YOUR HEALTH

You think you want to lose weight more than

anything? You think you would do anything to be slimmer? You probably already have all of the information you need to do this. So what's stopping you? Or what stops you once you've started?

Every day of my working life, I meet people who eat too much. They know they do, but they can't seem to stop. Sometimes it is nutritious food, sometimes it's not, but, whatever the case, they know they would be much better off if they ate less.

Often these people are seeing me because they want to lose weight and they are precious, intelligent people who don't understand why they do what they do. These people know what to eat and what not to eat to lose weight, yet they don't do it, even though they truly believe that they are desperate to lose weight.

There is a really big difference between eating two squares of chocolate and eating the entire block, between one biscuit (cookie) with a cup of tea in the evening and eating a dozen. We all know that eating too much makes us feel full and uncomfortable, but, worse, it usually drives us to say very unkind things to ourselves such as "I'm so useless, I have no willpower," and leads us to go to bed feeling guilty and sad and believing we will never be able to change. That belief that things are permanent is very destructive.

So what might be going on for someone who, even with good intentions, just can't stop eating?

Besides elevated cortisol caused by long-term stress, there may be other biochemical factors involved such as low progesterone, poor thyroid function, or blood sugar that surges and plummets. There are also likely to be emotional factors and core beliefs they probably aren't even aware of.

Don't worry about something until it becomes a problem. If it becomes a problem, then you can face it, but worrying about something that may never happen only serves to hurt you. As we now know, stress, whether it is real or perceived, may promote the production of excess cortisol. The ripple effect of a worry can very slowly and subtly change your metabolism to one of fat storage and leave your headspace full of sadness and withdrawn temperament. For some worry is at the heart of their rush. And it's the chemical signals created by your body, that your body believes will help you based on the information it is receiving, that are driving this.

ADRENAL FATIGUE

The next biochemical stage of stress that can occur, especially if the stress has been prolonged, may involve cortisol falling low. If you have had a high level of cortisol output for many, many years, your adrenal glands may not be able to stand the tension. They were never designed to sustain this kind of output and so they crash. In general terms, you "burnout." In more recent times, this has become known as adrenal fatigue, because the major symptom is a deep and unrelenting fatigue. Yet even with fatigue as the major symptom, what I have observed over the past decade is that not only are women beyond tired, at the same time they can also be wired. And when you are tired but wired, you desire deeply restorative sleep more than ever, yet it rarely happens, and your adrenal hormone production is usually at the heart of this. But remember from the introduction to this chapter about the endocrine system, that the pituitary gland is the master switch and so although treatment for adrenal fatigue usually involves a range of strategies that support the adrenals themselves, going one step further and assisting the pituitary can also be immensely powerful and highly beneficial to restoring your health and vitality.

The adrenal hormone cortisol is supposed to be high in the morning, and ideal amounts help you bounce out of bed. It plays a role in how vital you feel and helps the body combat any inflammatory processes that want to kick in. Stiffness is a key symptom of adrenal fatigue. For those with chronic stress, morning cortisol levels tend to be low, and, if 25 units is the ideal, with adrenal stress you may only get to 10 units. It can be very difficult to get out of bed with such low levels. By mid-afternoon, it will be at an all-time low, and you feel you need something sweet, something containing caffeine, or a nap to get you through your afternoon (this can also be the result of low blood sugar or poor thyroid function, explored in a later section). For an adrenally fatigued person, cortisol is nice and low in the evenings, but if you don't go to bed before 10:00pm, you will typically get a second wind, and it will be much harder for you to fall asleep if you're still up at midnight, partly due to the body's natural next adrenalin surge that tends to happen between 10:30pm and 11:30pm. The following graph illustrates this cortisol pattern.

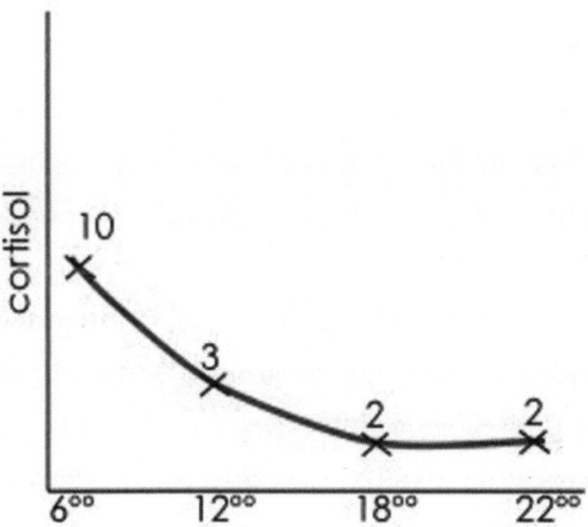

A typical cortisol profile of an adrenally fatigued person: *Note, particularly, the low waking cortisol and low midday reading.*

When cortisol drops low, it is likely that prior to this it was high (although not always), and body fat may have increased during this time. But just because it is low does not mean easy access to body fat burning due to cortisol's relationship to insulin, described earlier.

Additionally, the fatigue you feel with this biochemical picture may make exercise the least appealing thing on the planet to you. You actually feel worse after cardiovascular exercise when you are adrenally fatigued, whereas exercise typically energizes us. Frustration mounts because you believe that exercising and eating less are the only solutions to weight loss, yet you can't bring yourself to do either despite every good intention. Every time you eat something sweet, you eat too much, or another month goes past without much movement. When you reflect on this, you feel guilty, you might say mean things to yourself—and you may silently lose hope. You think "who cares?" now whenever you feel like eating something that won't really nourish you, and the not-so-great eating continues, especially an excess consumption of carbohydrates as you desperately search for energy. Your clothes keep getting tighter and this just adds to your stress. The vicious cycle is self-perpetuating.

Humans were never designed to sustain long-term stress, and our individual bodies cope with it in different ways. For some, adrenalin remains the dominant stress hormone all of their lives, while others may flip over into a more cortisol-dominant stress response. If the stress response doesn't truly switch off, there is the potential that the adrenals will eventually crash, and cortisol output is no longer optimum or elevated. It will be negligible. At its extreme, this is a condition called Addison's disease, yet if a person's cortisol level is extremely low but still falls just inside the "normal range," that person will be told that they are fine. They feel lousy but all the tests they have always come back "normal." They feel anything but normal, and people who know and love them will often comment that they are a shell of their former selves.

Cortisol can also be rather sinister in that it can interfere with your steroid (sex) hormone metabolism, your sleep patterns via its interference with melatonin, and also your mood via serotonin.

THE SEROTONIN-MELATONIN SEESAW

Is this your typical day? Healthy breakfast, mid-morning coffee, salad or sandwich for lunch... with probably something sweet to follow lunch but other than that, you are quite proud of yourself when you reflect on your food consumption so far for the day.

But I predict that many of you then fall into one of three categories later in the day. Do you:

1. Hit mid-afternoon and eat anything and everything in sight and then spend the rest of the day berating yourself after such a great start?
2. Get so busy during the afternoon that food does not enter your head until you arrive home and a glass of white wine and possibly some cheese and crackers allows you to let out a sigh of relief that the day is winding down?
3. Or is it neither of the above and the free-for-all starts after dinner, when you find yourself standing in front of the fridge or pantry saying to yourself "I want something. I don't know what it is that I want but I want something. And maybe it's in here!"

Perhaps all three of these scenarios apply to you! Never fear, a new understanding is near.

Options 1 and 2 are primarily about blood glucose. Option 3 describes "Miss Serotonin." Serotonin is our happy, calm, content hormone. It is the hormone that helps us feel like there is nothing for which we want in this world. It makes us content with our lot in life and helps keeps panic at bay. Melatonin is our sleep hormone and is responsible for sending us to, and keeping us, asleep. These hormones work antagonistically. That is, one goes up, the other goes down.

In our bodies we have what are called circadian rhythms, which govern a multitude of hormonal processes. These rhythms, coupled with fading sunlight, allow melatonin to rise, which, in turn, means serotonin must fall.

When a hormone that makes you feel happy, calm, and content (serotonin) decreases, it can create a noticeable sinking feeling or an irritation, a distinct change in mood even though nothing in the external world has changed. Five minutes before, you felt fine, yet now there is this nagging feeling that you want something; that something is not alright. There is a chance that a relatively lower level of serotonin as evening falls is partly why couples have conversations about "big ticket items" at this time of day. Our chemistry makes us feel like we want something and our brain tries to label what that might be. We usually don't find ourselves waking up and announcing that we absolutely must renovate the bathroom immediately! We keep those proclamations for evening and if you live with your significant other, they are more likely to be on the receiving end of a "more intense tone" describing what you have decided is missing from your life at this time of day! Of course that can be a good thing!

Hormones are powerful and they have the ability to not only alter your headspace and mood but also your food choices. Humans instinctively know that carbohydrate-rich foods promote serotonin production, which is partly why when the "I want something" syndrome hits, many women head for the pantry. You hope what you want is in there. Often, though, guilt is all you find.

Mornings can also prove a challenge for someone in this pattern. Melatonin is destroyed by sunlight, which is partly why when you go outside and exercise in the morning you tend to feel great all day. The melatonin plummets when the retina of your eyes is exposed to light and, as a result, your serotonin surges. On a day where you get up and expose your eyes to sunlight, with that hormonal profile, you can cope with anything. The flip side, though, is not so appealing. If you've gone to bed after midnight, not slept well, or both, you may not want to rise with the sun, or small children, as you don't feel rested. If you just wander out of bed sometime during the morning, your melatonin slowly seeps away, and your serotonin slowly rises. On such a day, you feel like you need a few coffees to get yourself going.

If this tale is ringing true for you, and the carb-fest in the evening feels out of control, the solution is not initially—or always—purely dietary.

Step one is to start getting up at the same time each morning and going outside and moving. If that is not possible because of your family situation, open the curtains and recognize a new day has dawned. Welcome the day with tai chi, a walk, some stretches, preferably something breath-focused. Commit to doing this for four weeks, every day, and observe if your evening carbohydrate cravings settle and notice if this helps any anxious feelings you may experience or that may intensify in the evenings. Your serotonin will love you for it.

PERCEPTIONS

As you can see, cortisol plays many roles in our body, and optimal levels are essential for us to be able to access body fat to burn it, to feel calm and content, have good energy, and keep inflammation and stiffness away.

Remember too that our perceptions play an enormous role in whether we are stressed or not. Sometimes it may be trauma in the past that takes a toll on your body. Even though you know in your mind you have dealt with it or moved on, your unconscious mind still wrestles with it. Or stress can be from comparatively "little" things. It is as if you have an itch that somehow gets scratched by your beloved, your children, your boss, or by random people. Our bodies go through everything with us, and despite our minds consciously moving on, sometimes our bodies are stuck in the past. Even more deeply, I hope that the messages on these pages will allow you to open yourself up to a new perspective on health, on food, on movement, on life, on feeling, on your beliefs, and, so importantly, on how calm and safe you feel in this world. There are some wonderful methods through which you can help shift your body and your emotions when you feel like you have cognitively processed the living daylights out of your stress, yet it still remains a challenge, your weight is still stuck, or you overreact to the undulations of life, where once you were more easily able to laugh at the calamity, the chaos, and the small stuff.

THE IMPORTANCE OF REST

You will see from the Solutions chapter later in the book that at the heart of all of my strategies to support you adrenally is the desire for you to rest and to rest well, in a restorative and revitalizing way. Rest must follow action for us to have optimal health, excellent fat burning, and the ability to remain calm, and very few of us these days truly rest, although we might believe we do. As outlined in the previous chapter, the parasympathetic nervous system is active when we truly rest. This is the "rest and repair" arm of our nervous system, but it can be dominated by the opposite arm of the nervous system, the sympathetic nervous system. The PNS also allows us to digest our food well and its activation is essential not only to feeling centred and calm, but to a tummy that isn't bloated after eating. Food is not supposed to bloat us yet a bloated stomach is a major complaint of more than 70 percent of women in the Western world. Calm is vital to optimal digestion, a topic covered in a later chapter. The following is an excerpt from an article I wrote for a magazine about the role of stress in illness which begins to explain some of the background to digestive system problems such as irritable bowel syndrome (IBS) and other health challenges.

The role of stress in illness

The human brain is made up of three integrated parts. The first brain is the brain stem or reptile brain. This is the survival brain. It controls all functions responsible for our survival, as an individual and as a species. It controls such things as hunger, thirst, heartbeat, breathing, digestion, immunity, and sex drive. It is the basic, primal part of us that is in all animals; give me food, give me shelter, let me reproduce!

This part of the brain also *initiates* the fight or flight stress response.

Our second brain is the limbic system or mammal brain. It is in all mammals and is composed of the amygdala, hippocampus, and thalamus. This is our emotional brain. It controls all functions related to emotional aspects of survival. It controls such things as memory, behaviour, pleasure, and pain responses, and our experience of all emotions. It *maintains* the fight or flight stress response.

The third brain is the cerebral cortex or human brain. Humans and some other mammals such as apes, dolphins, and whales have this brain, and it is our thinking brain. It controls such things as decision making, attention, awareness, language, judgment, reading, and writing. It is the centre of higher thought and it is *impaired* by the fight or flight stress response.

Every moment, our brain is assessing the world around us and asking the question: "Am I Safe?" This question is asked on all three levels: intellectually, emotionally, and from a survival perspective. If at any moment the brain determines you are in danger on any of these three levels, it sends out an alert to the body and the fight or flight stress response occurs. Mechanisms of survival are activated by the brain stem to prepare you to face the situation or run away. This occurs whether we are being chased by a tiger, sitting for an exam, seeing flashing lights in our rear view mirror, or being spoken to in an inappropriate way. It occurs any time the brain perceives "danger!"

The stress response in a nutshell looks like this. Adrenalin is released to provide more energy. The liver and muscles store a form of glucose called glycogen, and the body converts this back into glucose (sugar) to increase blood sugar levels and provide more energy. Blood pressure then rises, as does our pulse, to provide more oxygen to muscles. Our muscles tense to get us ready for action, and the pupils in our eyes dilate so we can see more in potentially less light. Immunity, digestion, and sexual functions all "turn off" as these three functions use energy not necessary for our immediate survival, and hunger and sex can also be distractions upon which we must not focus if we want to survive this perceived "threat" to our life.

All of these responses are appropriate to survive an attack from a tiger or any other danger. However, once the danger is gone and the stress is over, these body functions are designed to return to a state of balance. BUT! If during these stressful events the emotional brain or limbic system is involved (we feel fear, anger, resentment), it then sends a message to the brain stem to maintain the stress response to keep us safe, just in case such a situation ever happens again. Over time, this can develop into a chronic stress response even though we may not be able to recognise what led us to be stressed, given that often it is not an authentic threat to our life.

It is well recognised that "stress" plays a major role in the development of many illnesses as does the food we feed ourselves. Consider the list of stress physiology responses and it is immediately apparent that long-term, these are the Western world's most common chronic ailments.

The following list outlines some common ailments and their biochemical relationship to stress. They include:

- Adrenalin is released: anxiety
- Blood glucose increases: type 2 diabetes
- Blood pressure rises: hypertension
- Pulse increases: cardiac arrhythmia
- Muscles tense: neck and back pain
- Pupils dilate: far-sightedness
- Immunity downregulates: any immune related diseases
    - Digestion is downregulated: irritable bowel syndrome, constipation, indigestion
- Libido is downregulated: impotency, infertility

~~~~~~~~~~~~~~~~~~~~~~~~
~~~~~~~~~~~~~~~~~~~~~~~~

THE IMPORTANCE OF DIAPHRAGMATIC BREATHING

The breath is the only way we can consciously affect our ANS, which is why it is the cornerstone of all my adrenal support solutions. If you take nothing else away from this book I would like to encourage you with every ounce of my being to get a ritual in your day that allows you to focus on breathing well. It is not only key to shifting our chemistry from fat storage to fat burning, but it is the crucial strategy for cultivating calm. How can the breath drive such powerful shifts in your nervous system and your biochemistry?

The role of the ANS is to perceive the internal environment and, after processing the information in the central nervous system, regulate the function of your internal environment. The name "autonomic" implies that it is independent of the conscious mind. Think about a family of ducks and their newborn ducklings. Just like ducklings, the autonomic nervous system will always follow the leader, and the breath is the *only* part of the autonomic nervous system that can be controlled consciously. Your breath leads. Your body follows. Breathing dominates your autonomic nervous system, and because we breathe five thousand to thirty thousand times a day—or two to five hundred million times in your lifetime—it has the potential to influence you positively or negatively in many ways.

Nothing communicates to every cell of your body that you are safe better than your breath. If you breathe in a shallow way, with short, sharp inhalations and exhalations, then you communicate to your body that your life is in danger. You have just learnt about the cascade of hormonal events that follow such alarm and the role these hormones play in switching fat burning on or off. How you breathe is also a fast track to the symptoms of anxiety and, potentially, panic attacks, regardless of what led you to breathe in a shallow way in the first place, whether it was an event, a deadline, the perception of pressure, the "need" to rush, or the lifetime habit of your nervous system. Long, slow breathing that moves your diaphragm, communicates the opposite message to your body—that you are very safe. Nothing downregulates the production of fat storage stress hormones or the alarm signals within your body more powerfully.

Please practice diaphragmatic breathing, making sure your tummy moves in and out as you breathe, as opposed to just your upper chest. You can begin your breath by allowing the lower part of your tummy to expand and then imagine as the breath slowly continues that the expansion of your tummy has now extended into the area where you can feel your rib cage meet. Keep the slow inhalation going until your upper chest feels like it is pushing your ribs out at the sides of your body. Then pause, rather than hold your breath, and slowly allow the exhalation to begin in the reverse order of the inhalation with the top and side of the chest emptying first, followed by the middle of your abdomen and lastly your tummy. Please be kind and patient with yourself as this takes practice! You may feel like you are unable to get parts of your body to engage at first but, in time and with practice, the parts of you that have become disconnected will be thrilled to be back in touch.

At first you will more than likely need to schedule regularly breathing time slots into your day until it becomes your new way of breathing (unless you literally do need to escape from danger such as slamming your foot on the brake if another car suddenly drives out in front of you!). Make appointments with yourself to breathe. If it is peaceful each morning while you boil the kettle for the first time that day (to make your hot water with lemon of course!), instead of racing around and doing eighty jobs while the kettle boils, stand in your kitchen and breathe. Link breathing well to a daily routine, such as having a shower or to a particular hour of the day so that it quickly becomes a habit. Do it numerous times over the course of your day. Book a meeting into your calendar each afternoon at 3:00pm. If you work at a computer, have it pop up on the screen that it is time for your meeting with yourself to do twenty long, slow breaths. We keep appointments with other people, so be sure to keep the appointments you make with yourself. Take part in movement that facilitates a focus on the breath such as tai chi, qi gong, yoga, particularly restorative yoga, or walking quietly in nature. Pilates can also be useful, but I have found that it is highly dependent on your attitude while you are doing the session and also to some degree on the attitude of the instructor. For me personally, qi gong is how I choose to begin my day. It is not always easy to fit it in to a day with hourly meetings or appointments, but it is my habit now and has been for years. I had a period of time where I let this ritual go, however, and I soon learnt how crucial it is to set up my day with a restoration-focused session. My clarity, my sex hormone balance, and my vitality are not what I know they can be without it. So, please, schedule breathing focused periods into your day, and keep your appointments with yourself. The breath is the foundation pillar of calm and, therefore, of optimal health, and these practices allow us to still the stories that for many women fill their minds and are part of their source of stress.

THE IMPORTANCE OF LAUGHTER

Another free and powerful tool is laughter. If we see life as tough, full of hard work, pain, and drudgery, it will be precisely that. Humans have the ability to only see their perspective in the world, rather than the world as it truly is. We see the world through filters, yet we don't know they are there. I am not denying that life can be tough at times or that being honest with ourselves if we do feel down and out about life is not a good thing. The problem comes when we see the world this way and believe that it will never be any different. For then it won't be.

Think about it. A belief in the permanence of doom is dangerous for every hormonal signal in your body. Do your absolute best to shift your thinking to see life as an adventure, a journey, and a gift, full of opportunity, and a process through which you can contribute. Some of the greatest, most moving stories I have ever heard involved someone turning a horrific hardship into their greatest opportunity. Keep this in mind. Keep in mind, too, that you can choose to laugh at the calamity around you. I witnessed this recently when my dearest friend had her third baby and with him not even a day old, her deliciously spirited two-year-old sharing the delights of her day, countless well wishers chattering away, the hospital staff member wanting to clear the food tray away, and her two- year-old not being too thrilled about this… and all in one small room… my precious friend and her husband just shrugged and grinned at each other and laughed, internally clearly focused on the love in the room, rather than on anything else.

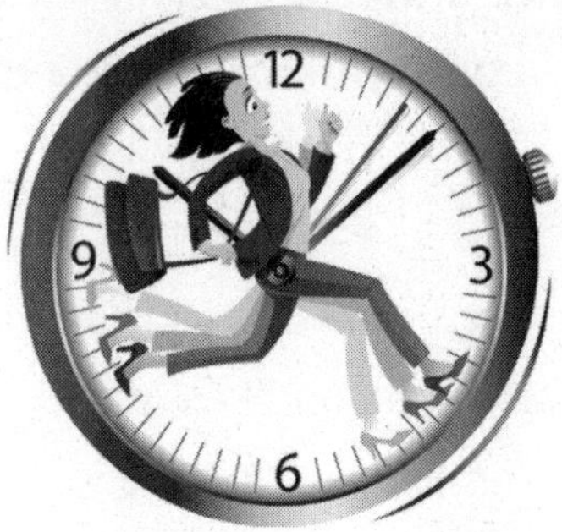

Chapter 3 Part 2

Your Ovaries and Your Sex Hormones: their role and impact on you in your rush

Another part of the endocrine system intimately involved in our capacity to feel calm, cope, and be happy involves the various glands and tissues that produce our sex hormones. In women, the ovaries are the main source of sex hormone production, however, both the adrenal glands and fat cells also make sex hormones. The body also contains tissues that produce hormones themselves but that are not sensitive to hormone levels in our body. The reason some tissues are hormone-sensitive and some are not relates to the presence of receptors for a particular hormone being present on that tissue. Let me explain.

HORMONES AND RECEPTORS: LIKE LOCKS AND KEYS

Just because your body may make a certain hormone, doesn't mean you get the lovely or the not so lovely effects of that hormone. For a hormone to illicit its effects, it has to bind to a receptor. The best way to imagine the way hormones interact with a receptor site is like a lock and a key. When they connect, you get the effects of the hormone. Breast tissue, for example, is highly sensitive to estrogen and progesterone, the two main female sex hormones, and this is the case because the breasts contain receptors for both of these hormones.

Sex hormones can be delicious substances that give you energy and vitality and yet they can also wreck havoc on your life. When it comes to a sense of calm, mental clarity, the ability to be patient and not make mountains out of molehills, fat burning, beautiful skin, as well as fertility, very few substances in our body impact us more than our sex hormones.

The main sex hormones we will cover in this chapter are estrogen, progesterone, and testosterone, with a particular focus on their role in body shape, size, fat burning, and inner peace, for when sex hormones are out of balance, this alone can have you feeling all pent up with far too many places to go.

CAN ESTROGEN MAKE YOU FRANTIC?

Estrogen is a feminine hormone (although men naturally make it in small amounts), and it plays numerous important roles in the human body, including ones associated with reproduction, promoting new bone growth, and supporting cardiovascular health. Challenges with estrogen occur, however, when there is too much of it compared to other hormones, progesterone in particular. Estrogen can also pose a problem if there is too much of one type of estrogen compared to other types of estrogen.

Estrogen is made by the ovaries of menstruating females, and small amounts are produced by fat cells and the adrenal glands. At menopause, ovarian production of hormones ceases.

The role of estrogen in the female body from a reproductive perspective is to lay down the lining of the uterus, which it does between days one and fourteen of a typical twenty-eight-day reproductive cycle, with day one of the cycle being the first day of menstruation. The estrogen lays the lining of the uterus down over these first fourteen days to prepare the female body for a conception if it takes place. Estrogen wants a menstruating female to fall pregnant every single month of her life, whether that is on her agenda or not! Remember, our bodies are completely geared for survival, and perpetuation of the human species is an enormous part of that survival process.

As a result of the biological imperative to conceive each month, estrogen ensures there is adequate body fat, as most females will not immediately know that they have fallen pregnant. In the event that the woman is a stick figure without much body fat, it is possible that a brand new foetus may not survive. To prevent this estrogen signals fat to be laid down in typically female areas, giving women a pear-like shape to better serve the childbirth process.

Estrogen is the hormone that makes female breasts bud at the first signs of puberty, it broadens hips, and it gives women their curves. It lays down fat on a woman's hips, bottom, and thighs, and is typically responsible for making the bottom half of a female body broader than the top half. Estrogen also, unfortunately, promotes fluid retention when it is in excess and this alone can be very stressful for a female… her clothes don't fit her the way she would like them to, and the last thing she wants when she feels like this is to be intimate, which for some women can lead to challenges with their significant relationship, adding another layer of stress to what is for many women an already overwhelming life.

FLUID RETENTION

I am convinced that many women "feel" fat when really they are either bloated or retaining fluid. As I said earlier, I have never once weighed a client and I don't encourage my clients to weigh themselves either. I do this for many reasons, but one is certainly because as hormone levels fluctuate over the month, so can the amount of fluid being retained until the hormones return to balance. Besides, when you weigh yourself, remember that all you are really doing is weighing your self-esteem. I have met thousands of women who can gain three kilos (six pounds) in a day, and to say that this messes with their mind is an understatement. If you get on the scales in the morning and weigh 70 kilograms (155 pounds), and, by the evening, you weigh 73 kilos (161 pounds), especially if you have eaten well and done some exercise that day, and even if you *haven't* eaten perfectly or exercised that day, it's easy to feel incredibly disheartened and wonder how on earth this could possibly happen. It can add an additional layer of stress to an already overloaded female mind… something else to worry and panic about.

Remember this: *it is not physically possible* to gain

three kilos (six pounds) of body fat in a single day. The only possible cause is fluid retention. Yet even though the logical part of the female mind knows this, seeing three extra kilos on the scales over the course of just a day, or even a week, will make most women, no matter how reasonable they are, feel fat, anxious, impatient, frustrated, and generally lousy. As an aside, are you more likely to make good food choices when you feel this way? Are you likely to want to be intimate with your partner when you feel fleshy and puffy and like there is not enough time in your day because if you are eating well and exercising and still gaining weight and well that must mean you have to find the time to do even more exercise and you don't know where on earth that time is going to come from because you already can't keep up… and that was all thought in such a hurry that now you are gulping for air!

There can be numerous factors behind fluid retention, too many to go into here, but in a nutshell, fluid retention can be driven by poor lymphatic flow, a congested liver from too many liver loaders, mineral deficiencies and imbalances, and poor progesterone production. From an energetic medicine perspective, I encourage you to think about who or what you may be holding on to that no longer benefits you. Perhaps it is a belief that no longer serves you, and your body is simply trying to wake you up to this and get you to change. So many of us fear change whether we realize it or not.

Estrogen can be another likely culprit when it comes to fluid in excess. It can also drive headaches, including migraines, increase blood clotting, decrease libido, and interfere with thyroid hormone production and, due to its relationship to progesterone, lead us to feel like we have to do everything with haste... big health consequences all because there is too much of one little hormone.

WHAT ROLE DOES PROGESTERONE PLAY?

Progesterone also plays a variety of roles in the human body. From a reproductive perspective, its job is to hold in place the lining of the uterus that estrogen has laid down between days one and fourteen of your cycle. If your body detects that a conception took place, the lining of the uterus needs to be maintained, rather than shed. As a result, progesterone levels begin to rise. If there is no conception, the lining of the uterus is not needed, and progesterone levels fall away, which initiates menstruation. When health is optimal, progesterone is the dominant sex hormone from just after mid-cycle onward until menstruation.

Biologically, progesterone has numerous other

roles, all pivotal to the *Rushing Woman's Syndrome* message. Progesterone is a powerful antianxiety agent, an antidepressant, and a diuretic, and it is essential if you are to access fat reserves to burn for energy. Without the right amounts of progesterone you will always burn your sugar, which may lead to your body having to break your muscles down for energy rather than accessing and burning fat stores. You may also have a tendency to an anxious or depressed mood and if you feel like you have a blessed life and yet you still feel low or like you complain, add guilt to that emotional cocktail and a degree of confusion about what is really bothering you. You can see how layer upon layer of physical and emotional stress can form.

The relationship between sex hormones and stress hormones is fascinating and powerful, and it's where an aspect of the physical, biochemical approach of *Rushing Woman's Syndrome* is focused. And this is because nine out of ten women who see me for consultations enjoy positive changes in their body and their health when we address this.

THE RELATIONSHIP BETWEEN STRESS AND SEX HORMONES

Estrogen is the dominant sex hormone between day one and day fourteen of the menstrual cycle.

As described earlier, its job is to lay down the lining of the uterus and make sure there is enough body fat in the event of conception. For the first half of the menstrual cycle, a relatively small amount of progesterone is made from our adrenal glands. For the sake of this description, let's call the amount 2 units. Remember, the reproductive role of progesterone is to hold the lining of the uterus in place with the additional biological functions of it being an antianxiety agent, antidepressant, diuretic, and fat burner.

However, as you now understand from the previous section, your adrenal glands are also where you make your stress hormones, namely adrenalin and cortisol. Adrenalin communicates to every cell of your body that your life is being threatened, even though all you may have done is had an argument with your beloved, and he spoke to you inappropriately because he felt like a failure at the time. Men usually don't behave well when they subconsciously create a meaning of failure as an emotion—which could come from a question you asked (without any loaded meaning behind it) or a focus on his bank balance that is not where he "needs" it to be to feel safe. Women typically behave in a way they (or those around them) don't enjoy so much when they feel rejected. This does not excuse poor behaviour, but rather offers an explanation to promote understanding. My point is to highlight that both physical (e.g. caffeine) and emotional (perception of pressure or creating a meaning of rejection from an argument) processes can drive adrenalin production and communicate that danger is nigh.

As you now understand, when you are internally rattled, cortisol communicates to every cell of your body that there is no food left in the world and, as a result, it wants your body to break muscle down and store fat. Even though food is, in fact, abundant for you, and your cortisol production is likely to be coming from the areas of your life about which you feel uncertain, such as relationships, finances, or even what others might think of you, your body thinks there must be a flood, famine, or a war, as this was the only long-term stress humans historically experienced.

Since your body links progesterone to fertility, if your body's perception is that your life is under threat and that there is no food left in the world, the last thing it wants is for a woman to conceive, so it shuts down adrenal progesterone production. Estrogen and cortisol, both signalling fat storage and continuing stress remain, while you've lost the counterbalancing hormone that keeps you calm and helps burn fat and get rid of excess fluid!

I believe this situation alone is a modern day, monumental shift in female chemistry, and it can torment a woman's emotional and physical well-being. This shift plays an enormous role in both why you rush and the perception of the need to rush; another vicious cycle. A female can go from feeling happy, healthy, balanced, and energized, with great clarity of mind and an even mood, to having a foggy brain and feeling either overly anxious about things she cannot name or utterly exhausted as a result of this shift to excess estrogen and cortisol coupled with low progesterone. Physically she may feel puffy, heavy, bloated and full of fluid, with a sense that her clothes are getting tighter by the minute. And that is just the first half of the cycle!

A menstruating female ovulates around day fourteen of her cycle, and there are numerous hormonal changes that occur to drive ovulation. Once the egg has been released from the ovary, a crater remains on the surface of the ovary where the egg popped out. This crater is called the corpus luteum, and it's where the bulk of a woman's progesterone is made. Progesterone is designed to peak on day twenty-one of a twenty-eight day cycle at around 25 to 40 units. If conception takes place, progesterone levels need to climb to continue to hold the lining of the uterus in place. Once the placenta has formed by week 12 of gestation, progesterone levels climb to around 300 to 400 units. Pregnancy is the time when a woman has the highest level of circulating progesterone. Once a woman has birthed the placenta, however, her progesterone level plunges from 350 to zero! It is fortunate that birth brings on some other feel good hormones, such as oxytocin (explored later), although they tend to be more short-lived.

Historically, babies were welcomed into extended families and communities. Today, a more common scenario (not the only scenario) is a hospital birth followed by a new mother at home alone with her newborn during the day while her partner must continue to work to pay the mortgage and other bills. If there are challenges in their relationship or challenges caused by the needs of other children, financial stress, ill or aging parents, an ill newborn or simply one who won't sleep, the new home environment with baby can be highly stressful. Another stressful scenario I've heard described thousands of times is one where a new mother has made what she thought would be a welcomed transition (temporarily or permanently) from a corporate career to staying at home with her baby, but is now second-guessing her decision. The guilt and confusion around this scenario can be overwhelming. Such scenarios do not promote the restoration of adrenal progesterone levels, as the body is so busy making stress hormones that it is not "safe" for the new mum to make the fertility-linked progesterone. Remember, progesterone is one of the most powerful antianxiety and antidepressant substances the body makes. On the other hand, if Mum and baby do have support, and the new mom doesn't feel she is alone with her new precious bundle, whether this is simply due to the mother's beliefs, attitudes, and perceptions, or her actual physical support from other people, then adrenal progesterone levels are far more likely to be restored, and her chemistry is all the better for it.

If conception does not take place during a menstrual cycle, maintaining the lining of the uterus is no longer necessary and progesterone levels fall, allowing a female to bleed. However, something that is so common today is what is known as "luteal phase insufficiency," where ovarian progesterone production is poor and a peak of 25 units in the second half of the cycle is not reached. Progesterone may be the dominant hormone from day 16 to day 18 of the cycle, but it falls away too soon (it is supposed to be dominant from just after mid-cycle at around day 14 until around day 27), and estrogen becomes dominant leading into the menstrual bleed.

This estrogen dominance is the biochemical basis of pre-menstrual syndrome (PMS) which causes grief for the woman as well as for most people around her! When PMS occurs it can be because estrogen is dominant for all but two or three days of a twenty-eight day cycle, meaning that progesterone gets no time to rule the roost, and a woman misses out on all its delicious stress-busting, calm-inducing and fat-burning qualities.

WHAT HAPPENS WHEN ESTROGEN IS DOMINANT?

The typical symptoms of low progesterone include:

- Premenstrual migraine
- PMS-like symptoms
- Irregular or excessively heavy periods
- Anxiety and nervousness
- A feeling like you can't get your breath past your heart

The typical symptoms of estrogen dominance (which usually also involves low progesterone—but not always) include:

- Irregular periods or excessive vaginal bleeding
- Bloating/fluid retention
- Breast swelling and/or tenderness
- Decreased libido

- Mood swings, most often irritability, easy to anger, and/or depression
- Weight gain, especially around the abdomen and hips
- Cold hands and feet
- Headaches, particularly premenstrually
- Tendency to yellow-tinged skin

This is the most common hormonal imbalance I see in menstruating women. The significant excess of estrogen being made within the female body, combined with increased estrogen in our environment (food and chemicals such as pesticides), appear to be affecting our endocrine (hormonal) systems in literally life-changing ways.

It is essential to discern whether a woman is suffering from symptoms of estrogen dominance caused by excess estrogen or by significantly low progesterone levels. For the latter it would mean that adrenal and/or ovarian production of progesterone is poor. This person may have optimal estrogen levels, yet they are challenged with their periods and/or their body fat due to low progesterone levels. The hormones that signal ovulation to occur are made by the pituitary gland so, again, optimal progesterone production is reliant on good communication between the pituitary and the ovaries.

Another extremely common scenario is one of estrogen excess. This can come about through excessive environmental exposures, including use of the oral contraceptive pill, hormone replacement therapy, plastics, and pesticides. Another significant basis for estrogen excess is estrogen recycling as a result of poor estrogen detoxification by the liver. In a nutshell, the liver decides whether to excrete or recycle estrogen. The liver prioritizes what it needs to detoxify and because the body makes estrogen itself, it is not a high priority to clear it from the body. A woman can have this month's estrogen circulating as well as last month's and even estrogen from numerous previous months. Even the best progesterone producer cannot balance and keep up with so much estrogen.

An additional estrogen-dominant hormonal picture is a combination of both the descriptions above of poor progesterone production and recycled estrogen. If we took better care of our liver, this would be far less common in the Western world. As I love to say, these things have become common, but they are not normal. Women are not supposed to get PMS. Your period is supposed to just turn up... no extreme mood swings, no pain, no pre-menstrual migraines... just menstruation.

The following is an article I wrote for breast cancer

awareness month. The brief I was given was to write about what makes breasts healthy. Some of it repeats information I have included earlier and also information from *Accidentally Overweight*, but I left it here to remind you of how vitally important these factors are and because breast cancer tragically is the leading cancer killer among women between the ages of twenty and fifty-nine in high-income countries, the same population affected by PMS and the perceived need to rush.

Healthy Breasts

When it comes to breast health, there is so much we now understand that contributes to the creation and maintenance of healthy breast tissue. Empowering women to take charge of this incredibly important aspect of their health is vital to the future of all women, and education must begin at a young age. Part of the challenge is deciphering fact from fiction or fad, so let's explore what we know creates healthy breasts.

Hormones, Stress, and the Liver

Although the hormone estrogen does some wonderful things for our health, too much of it or too much of a particular type of estrogen has been linked to some breast cancers. What is important to explore, when it comes to our hormones, is, why is estrogen so much more of a problem now as opposed to a time in the not so distant past? Part of the explanation lies in the production of stress hormones, and part of the explanation lies with the excretion of estrogen following liver detoxification of this substance.

When we are stressed, we make either, or both, of our two dominant stress hormones, namely adrenalin or cortisol. Adrenalin communicates to every cell of your body that your life is in danger, and cortisol tells your body that food is scarce. As a result, levels of another sex hormone called progesterone, which has been shown to be protective against breast cancer (except those that are progesterone receptor positive), falls through the floor as the body links progesterone to fertility. If the body believes that your life is in danger and that there is no more food left in the world, the last thing it wants for you is a pregnancy. And so begins part of the problem with estrogen; it is dominant in comparison to progesterone. This situation may also arise from synthetic forms of estrogen, such as from the oral contraceptive pill (OCP) or hormone replacement therapy (HRT).

The second scenario to consider involves the excretion pathway of estrogen out of the body. Once a molecule of estrogen has done its job for a specific time, it is transported to the liver where it has to be transformed so that it can be excreted. There are two phases to this detoxification process. Over the years, the workload of the liver in its second stage of this cleaning process can get clogged, just like traffic on a motorway. Where once substances flew through the liver at 100 kilometres per hour (62 miles per hour), they now crawl through at 20 kilometres per hour (12 miles per hour). When this process becomes terribly overloaded from years of too much alcohol, caffeine, refined sugars, trans fats, or the by-products of bowel congestion (a tendency to constipation), the estrogen will undergo its first stage of change, but there is no room on the second stage highway so the estrogen is released by the liver back into the blood stream. Your body is then faced with the new estrogen it continues to make from your ovaries (if you are still menstruating) and your fat cells, as well as the recycled form. It is this recycled form of estrogen that has been found to be up to four hundred times higher in women with estrogen sensitive breast cancer.

Looking after your precious liver is one of the best steps you can take to ensure your breast tissue remains healthy. Sadly, many women regularly overconsume alcohol, and it is this *regular, overconsumption* that is undeniably linked to the development of cystic breast tissue and breast cancer. Women need to get real about how much they are drinking. Heart organizations around the world suggest that two standard drinks per day (equivalent of two 100 millilitre [100 mL is the equivalent of 3.4 fl oz.] glasses of wine) with two days off each week is acceptable. Cancer research suggests, however, that if you have a family history of breast cancer, there is no safe level of alcohol consumption. That is a massive statement. If alcohol is something you enjoy, don't drink it daily. Save it for special occasions. Sparkling water with fresh lemon or lime can be a great, refreshing alternative.

Caffeine—coffee in particular—has also been found to play a role in the creation of denser, cystic breast tissue. On the other hand, green tea has consistently been shown in numerous studies to be protective against many types of cancers, breast cancer included. Most people are astounded at the changes in their breasts when they take a break from coffee and alcohol. As a woman living in the same world as all of you, a world with plenty of alcohol and caffeine on offer, I challenge you to take a break from these substances no matter how much you love or depend on them. Do it for one week, one little week out of your big long life. Once you've done that, do it for two. Or better still, omit them for one or two menstrual cycles and notice how different your breasts feel.

Diet and exercise

When it comes to the aspects of our

diets that are essential for healthy breast tissue, vegetables and fruits head the list. All of the cruciferous vegetables (Brassica family) have potent anticancer properties. Broccoli, in particular, contains sulphoraphane, a compound that helps the body begin to eliminate carcinogenic substances from the body in as little as ten days after it is included in the diet on a daily basis. It also keeps estrogen from binding to and stimulating the growth of breast cancer cells, a vital step in keeping breast tissue healthy. The great news, too, is that sulphoraphane survives cooking. Eat broccoli ladies!

Eat fruits and vegetables that are also rich in beta-carotene. On average, women with breast cancer tend to have lower levels of beta-carotene in their blood, although researchers cannot say whether this is a cause or a result of the disease. A small-scale study in Italy found that beta-carotene given with other, related carotene compounds increased the tumour-free period among women who already had breast cancer. The safest and most effective way to maintain healthy levels of beta-carotene is to consume five or more servings of dark-green, yellow, or orange vegetables and citrus fruits daily. We must eat our vegetables every day. No excuses!

Make an effort to minimize your consumption of fried foods and charcoal-grilled meats. Also, there is significant evidence to suggest that reducing our consumption of animal foods and basing our diet mostly on plant-based foods is incredibly beneficial to breast health and the prevention of breast cancer.

A growing body of literature suggests that insulin resistance is now a contributing factor in numerous cancers. Insulin is a hormone that can behave like a growth factor. It encourages all cells to grow: fat cells, healthy normal cells, and cells that may be precancerous or cancerous. The best way to limit insulin production in the body is to never base a meal purely on carbohydrates. The only carbs humans traditionally ate were those from berries, legumes, and pulses (we might call these lentils and beans, such as garbanzo beans or chickpeas). Today, we are faced with a barrage of highly processed foods, rich in sugars and starches. Limit your intake of these. We also tend to forget that most alcoholic drinks are packed with sugar.

Remember it is what you do every day that will have the most impact on your health, not what you do sometimes. It is not about going without; it is about getting real about what you, as a woman, already know to be true. You know better than anyone when you have too much of a particular substance in your diet... whether it is alcohol, coffee, or sugar. Make the changes you know you need to make now.

You will give your breasts a great chance of remaining healthy in the process.

Lastly, move your body. The benefits of regular movement are well documented for many areas of our health, including a reduction in insulin levels and body fat, both of which, in excess, have been linked to unhealthy breast tissue.

Nutrients for healthy breasts

Most of us have heard about the importance of iodine for optimal thyroid function and in the prevention of goitre. What we hear very little about is how vital iodine is to breast health. The breasts concentrate iodine as do the ovaries, and studies have shown that a form of estrogen associated with breast cancer can be produced by the ovaries in an iodine-deficient state. This has been shown to be reversible once iodine levels are optimal again. Use a salt that contains iodine, add seaweeds to cooking, or take a supplement.

Also of great consequence to breast health is our dietary intake and ratio of essential fatty acids. These are predominantly found in oily fish, flaxseeds, walnuts and pecans, evening primrose oil, and borage oil. It can be difficult to eat enough of these vital fats on a daily basis, so a good supplement combining at least fish or flax with evening primrose oils can be a great addition to your daily diet. Start with two capsules in the morning and two at night or one to two tablespoons of the liquid oil.

Another mineral that is essential for healthy breast tissue is magnesium and, coupled with selenium, these nutrients have been shown to reduce the incidences of new breast cancers. Green, leafy vegetables are high in magnesium, while brazil nuts are rich in selenium. Eat them daily, or take a supplement.

Vitamin C is one of the most important nutrients when it comes to so many aspects of our health. The list of wonderful activities vitamin C performs in the body is almost endless. It helps keep the immune system responding appropriately to stimuli, and hastens white blood cell response times.

Vitamin B6 has also been extensively researched when it comes to breast health. Eggs are a good source, as are bananas and avocados.

Herbs for healthy breasts

Two of my favourite herbs work on the adrenal glands. These are rhodiola and the Ginseng family. Both herbs are considered to be adaptogens, which means they help the body adapt to stressors by fine-tuning the stress response. These herbs tend to have a calming effect on the nervous system, which in turn promotes appropriate sex and stress hormone production rather than extremes.

Other herbs that have been shown to be useful in creating healthy breast tissue are those that promote liver detoxification and bile production from the gall bladder. Bile is essential for the appropriate excretion of any fat-soluble substances from the body, including cholesterol and estrogen. Useful herbs include St Mary's thistle, Globe artichoke, Bupleurum, and Schisandra.

Minimize exposure to...

The final thing you need to know about the creation and maintenance of healthy breast tissue involves the things that are best kept to a minimum. Minimizing our exposure to growth factor-like substances, including insulin, may be an important aspect of maintaining healthy breast tissue. Dairy products naturally contain growth factors, since the milk is designed to grow a 40 kilogram (88 pound) baby calf into a 900 kilogram (almost 2000 pound) beast. The growth factors naturally present in milk and milk products drive this growth. Humans, however, aren't designed to grow at these rates. If milk must be consumed, sheep and goats are smaller animals so their milks tend to drive slower, smaller growth rates. Alternatively, nut milks contain no growth factors. For people with diabetes who need insulin, eating a diet that limits the need for insulin without, however, compromising blood glucose levels is important.

There is also a growing and very concerning body of evidence that points at the importance of minimizing our exposure to plastics and pesticides. They disrupt our endocrine (hormonal) systems and can mimic estrogen. Recent research out of the United States shows that a large percentage of girls aged eight have hit puberty, leading to longer estrogen production over their lifetime. Furthermore, fewer pregnancies also lead to relatively more time spent in estrogen-dominant states. Researchers suggest that poor diet, lack of exercise, high body fat, and exposure to plastics are the likely culprits for the earlier onset of menstruation. We can make a really big difference to our health and our children's health by getting these lifestyle factors on track.

~~~~~~~~~~~~~~~~~~~~~~~~

REPRODUCTIVE SYSTEM CONDITIONS

There are numerous reproductive conditions that involve poor progesterone production or estrogen dominance in some way, and both of these scenarios have different effects on how a woman feels and functions. Polycystic ovarian syndrome (PCOS) is one of these conditions.

Polycystic ovarian syndrome

In PCOS, the eggs in the ovaries ripen on the surface of the ovary but are not released. They harden
~~~~~~~~~~~~~~~~~~~~~~~~

and form cysts (hence the name of the condition). As you now understand, to obtain optimal progesterone levels crucial for calm and fat burning, ovulation is essential, since the majority of your monthly progesterone is made by the corpus luteum.

Other hormones are also involved in PCOS. The pituitary gland makes luteinizing hormone (LH) and follicle stimulating hormone (FSH). Just prior to day fourteen of a typical cycle, both hormones increase, but in PCOS both of these hormones from the pituitary gland tend to flatline. Testosterone, the dominant male sex hormone, also tends to be higher in women with PCOS.

The LH and FSH hormonal profile of an ideal menstrual cycle is illustrated in the figure below while the profile of someone with PCOS is represented in the second figure.

Normal Menstrual Cycle

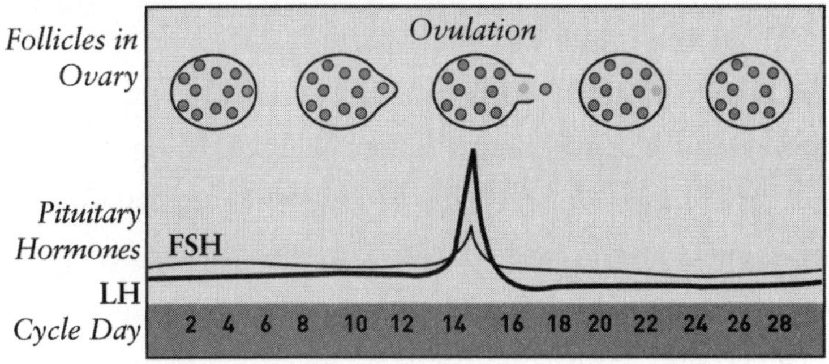

Ideal LH and FSH peaks generating ovulation:
Both LH and FSH peak to drive ovulation.

PCOS

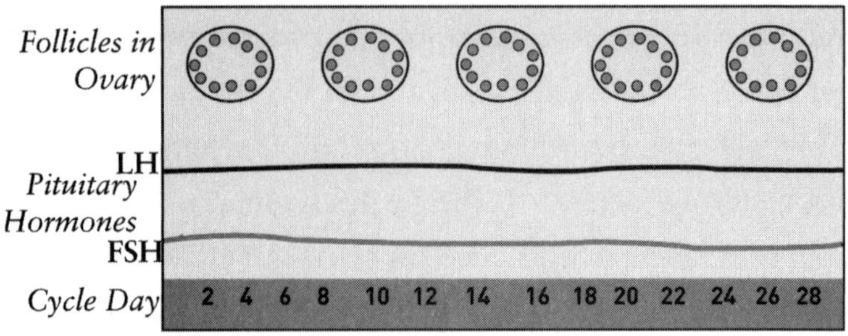

A Typical PCOS LH and FSH Profile:
Both LH and FSH tend to flatline in PCOS with LH levels remaining consistently elevated.

REPRODUCTIVE CONDITIONS: BIOCHEMISTRY, BELIEFS AND FEMININITY

When it comes to challenges with the reproductive system or hormones, I find exploring not only the biochemistry but also the subconscious beliefs and behaviours for each individual very useful and often the gateway to real change and health improvements. This is nowhere clearer than in PCOS.

From a hormonal perspective, in PCOS, not only do the two pituitary hormones, LH and FSH, tend to flatline, but the other female sex hormones of estrogen and progesterone tend to be low, while testosterone tends to be on the high end of normal or elevated out of the normal range. With most other reproductive system health conditions, estrogen tends to be high. There are a number of theories about why estrogen tends to be low in PCOS, including genetics, poor transformation of cholesterol into estrogen and an altered hypothalmic-pituitary-adrenal (HPA) axis, which is system that links those three glands via hormonal communication. Stress impacts significantly on HPA axis function and in some women with PCOS, it is theroised that a possible outcome of overt or silent stress may be the formation of cysts on the ovary. I investigate all of these factors in clients and encourage you to know where you sit biochemically with all of these hormones.

I also explore all health conditions with which I am presented from an emotional and a meta-physical perspective to help an individual gain more insight into any beliefs that may be behind their health condition for I have found that it is often the combination of sorting both the biochemistry and the beliefs that harbours great results.

Think about this. There is nothing more feminine than our ovaries; men don't have them. With PCOS, however, it is as if the ovaries have gone deaf. The pituitary gland has been calling out to the ovaries in an attempt to alert them to release an egg, the most feminine process that goes on inside a woman. For the ovaries to no longer hear the call from the pituitary, there could be a very silent, unconscious belief from somewhere in this person's world that they have to behave like a man in order to receive appreciation, connection, or love. Somewhere in their past, more masculine behaviour has been rewarded.

Women have shown they can match men in every arena. But there are types of work that, even today, are still more male dominated. I have met countless women, working in what were previously more male-dominated roles in particular, whose hormonal profiles have taken on a decidedly masculine appearance. These women are incredibly capable. The problem, however, lies in their (usually unconscious) beliefs about how they have to be in order to perform and achieve and, without realising it, therefore be "loved." Most often, they do not even realize that they are thinking or behaving "like a man" until we explore what that looks like. It is the mental approach to the work not the work or job itself that tends to be masculine.

Please don't get me wrong. I am not suggesting all professional women have got or will get PCOS, nor am I suggesting that to be a woman and have a highly successful career means you have behaved like, or in the future will have to behave like, a man. What I am simply wanting to point out is that your *attitude*, your *perception* of who you have to be, how you must behave, what you have to achieve or do to get approval is likely to be based on more masculine beliefs and behaviours and it may not have ever struck you, that you even believe this let alone that there is another way; that in fact you don't need to "do" (masculine) anything to be loved. You simply need to "be" (feminine).

Our chemistry is ancient. What we ask of our bodies today is entirely different from what we asked of them even fifty years ago. On the one hand, it is truly remarkable what our bodies can do: work sixteen-hour days sitting at a desk, eat more processed rather than nutrient-dense food, while we constantly think up solutions to challenges presented during the day, meet deadlines, juggle phone calls, crises, and complaints, and hopefully also celebrate a few things. And this is just the tip of the iceberg. On the other hand, we are so very far removed from the way humans have lived for 149,950 years that I believe the human body is rebelling, and one of the most obvious areas is women's reproductive health, including fertility.

If this rings true for you, explore ways you can bring more feminine rituals into your life. What do you associate with femininity? If you need to be "masculine" at work, do it, but bring compassion into your heart and soften your gaze when you're there. No one will know this is what you've done. Don't look at the work on your desk and tense up.

Instead, notice the work on your desk and take a long slow breath that moves your belly when you inhale. Feel, and I mean really feel, really notice how tension feels in your body. And then relax into it. Only you know you've done this. The feminine feels and so many women have become so detached from their body that they are unaware of how they truly feel in the body. Your productivity and contribution will still be enormous and perhaps even more than what you found possible from a state of tension. Think about "creating" instead of "producing." In emotional medicine, the ovaries are the seats of creativity. Just that shift in language is more feminine and can be helpful.

When you come home, as often as you can, be a complete girl! Light a candle and notice the fragrance. Dance around your house to music you love! Have a bubble bath. Giggle with the children or at a comedy. Read a girly book if that appeals to you. Make a pot of herbal tea after dinner in a teapot you love, and turn it into an "occasion." Notice the design of the pot and cup, the fragrance, and how you feel taking care of yourself. Masculinity (not men, but masculine energy) would never do this. But a man embracing his feminine would, just to point out the difference.

Please understand, this not an anti-feminist

concept. Addressing the biochemistry of PCOS is of enormous importance to getting health results, including calm. I simply wanted to highlight the incredible benefit I have witnessed when women embrace their feminine essence in more areas of their lives. And feminine rituals are a beautiful place to start. I encourage all women with PCOS to explore what they perceive their fathers expected of them or whom they had to be to "earn" his love. And you will more than likely see that this is at the heart of why you do much of what you do and that that is OK. Only it is no longer OK if it is hurting your health. And then breathe, soften, and relax.

PUBERTY

Some girls breeze through this time of transition without much change in their moods or their bodies, while, for others, an anxiety or even a darkness can set in. Estrogen is the first female sex hormone to be made in any great quantity in a girl's body. As beautiful as estrogen can be as a hormone, it can wreck havoc when it is present in substantial amounts for the first time ever, in young female bodies that do not yet have sufficient progesterone being made to counterbalance its effects.

Prior to menstruation beginning, estrogen is being made causing the breasts to bud and promoting the growth of pubic hair. It also begins to drive fat storage for all of the reasons outlined earlier. Some girls appear to be more "fleshy" for a time just prior to menarche, indicating estrogen is fulfilling its role.

Because progesterone is a powerful antianxiety agent and an antidepressant, if it is slow to initiate, a girl who was once bouncy, bright, full of energy, and interested in things, can become flat or anxious in her moods and distant in her relationships. If her periods do begin and they are irregular and/or heavy and painful, to the extent she is unable cope with school or life in general, she will often be encouraged to go on the oral contraceptive pill. It is important to understand two things here. One is the way the contraceptive pills work and the second is the biochemical process that occurs at the onset of menstruation.

Firstly, the pill is successful at preventing pregnancy because it shuts down the ovarian production of hormones. The number of women of all ages I meet who have no idea how this powerful medication works astounds me. I am neither pro-pill nor anti-pill; I simply want people to make informed choices. I will say it again. The pill shuts down ovarian production of hormones, and the body relies entirely on the synthetic version of hormones being supplied by the tablet. Substances in patented medications, such as the pill, must be at least ten percent different from the form the body naturally makes. They are not identical to the form created by the body.

With the ovaries shut down, the adrenal production of progesterone becomes even more important, yet is unlikely to be optimal given what can be a stressful time around the onset of menstruation and, for some girls, the increase in body fat for the first time. Never never *ever* comment on an adolescent girl's changing shape and size by encouraging her to eat less. That stresses her more as she may feel like she is letting you down when she doesn't do it; it doesn't matter whether you are her parent, teacher, or friend. Explain that, for a while, hormones can change our shapes, and eating nutritious food and staying active are the most important things to do to stay healthy. Tell her not to worry about it and demonstrate your love for her with your actions not just words. With less stress, which may be caused by her private perception of how her life is, which may gently be explored, her progesterone is more likely to kick in, and her body shape and size will sort itself out. Some areas that can be useful to explore in this situation is an adolescent female's perception of academic pressure and her perception of what it may mean to a family member if she "fails" (which may mean not coming out on top of her class in some cases). Exploring what her "friends" are saying at school can also prove insightful.

The second issue that needs to be explored is the biochemistry associated with the onset of menstruation. This is the first time in a girl's life that her pituitary gland sends signals to her ovaries. For approximately the first five years, the chemical messengers released by the pituitary follow a road to the ovaries that looks like a goat track, meaning that it is a path that sometimes reaches a destination (in this case the ovaries) and sometimes winds up heading off into no-man's-land. In other words, sometimes the pituitary signals miss their mark. After about five years, this pathway, if it has been allowed to become established, behaves like a five-lane highway. The route is clear, straight, and unhindered.

What I see, though, repeatedly are girls who have gone onto the pill to manage irregular or very heavy periods rather than for contraception, shortly after menstruation begins. If sport is a big issue or school is being missed due to severe period pain, then perhaps there may be occasions when the use of the pill is appropriate, and I certainly do not want to illicit feelings of guilt in parents or daughters in this area. But the pill simply masks the truth. If a girl stays on the pill long-term, the five-lane highway is never established. She will then come off the pill in adulthood, potentially wanting to have babies, but her pituitary has no history of communicating with her ovaries. It is a lot to ask our ovaries to suddenly wake up when we have suppressed their function for an extended period of time.

I cannot encourage you enough to get to the bottom of *why* the pain or the irregularity occurs in the first place. Before deciding about whether or not the pill is the best choice, explore other options and seek ways to change the hormonal imbalance that may be present, or at least give the pituitary-ovary pathway time to become established.

As far as moods are concerned, what breaks my heart is seeing a young woman start menstruating, with very heavy periods and some weight gain despite still eating well, disappear into her mind with her own private focus on sad thoughts and an anxiety that often comes out with nervous type behaviours, such as picking at her finger nails. This can be the first time ever that a girl experiences a tendency to depression or anxiety and her family is often bereft and concerned at the change in their girl. The most common intervention in this situation is the prescription of the pill. But because the pill does not correct what is likely to be slow-starting or insufficient progesterone, the young woman's mood doesn't lift, despite her periods now being regulated (by the pill). So she is encouraged by well-meaning adults to take an antidepressant. She is not even halfway through her teens, and she is on two incredibly potent, powerful medications.

There are times when conventional medicine is lifesaving, and I am not suggesting it be avoided at all costs, especially not at the cost of precious human life. What I am encouraging, initially, is the balancing of estrogen and progesterone through natural methods with the support of an experienced health professional. Counselling at the same time may also be incredibly beneficial to assist with the new darker thoughts that may have arisen. My holistic approach means also discussing any fears this young woman may have about her perception of what it means to be an adult woman. It can be the first time she ever feels fleshy, puffy, or bloated, and, to a young mind influenced so heavily by popular magazines, it is easy to understand why she can think she is fat when all she is, is estrogen dominant. As I said earlier, it is not physically possible to gain three kilos (six pounds) of fat in one day. It is most likely due to fluid and, given the diuretic action of progesterone, a deficiency of this vital hormone is one of the likely culprits of this young woman's fleshy feelings.

At its simplest level, menopause is the ceasing of the ovarian production of hormones. But production continues from the adrenal glands and fat cells. However, as explained earlier, many women now make insufficient amounts of progesterone from their adrenals because of chronic stress. In my opinion, this is such a powerful factor in whether a woman breezes through menopause with few or no debilitating symptoms, or whether the heat and the sleeplessness become overwhelming. If you are approaching menopause, I cannot encourage you enough to ensure your adrenal function is optimal. Apply the adrenal care techniques described in the solutions chapter of this book, using breathing strategies and herbal support, combined with lifestyle changes where possible.

If you are post-menopausal, I also can't encourage you enough to address adrenal health and liver health, strategies for which are also in the solutions section. Heat from the body can certainly be due to low estrogen levels or liver congestion. If I meet a client who has tried all sorts of natural estrogen therapies and used herbs that have an estrogenic action such as Black cohosh, and they are still overwhelmingly hot and suffering debilitating hot flushes (flashes), I will treat their liver.

Remember that in traditional circles, menopause is a time when wisdom begins to flow constantly. Trust what you already know inside of you when it comes to your health. You innately know better than anyone else what is best for you. Seek guidance from health professionals, but apply only what makes sense to you.

MENSTRUATION AND REST

Many women already know what I am about to share with you. Perhaps this is something you have observed in yourself and that is, that menstruation can be a time of soothing, stilling calm, a natural bliss. With some care and attention from you, this time can become your own natural, inbuilt zone to de-stress.

In our 24/7 lifestyles it is more important than ever to create islands of calm… timeout in which to release tension and simply "be" for a while. Just as we can't go without sleep for too long, your psyche cannot push on for too long without some quality downtime. The time you menstruate is the classic cyclic downtime due to the hormonal pattern and the energetics that exists at that time. The hormone involved is called oxytocin, also known as the love hormone, as it engenders feelings of love, calm, and belonging. It is released during sexual activity, birth and breastfeeding, as well as when we are touching, hugging, and sharing a meal. Orgasm causes oxytocin levels to rise from three to five times higher than baseline, creating feelings of closeness and tenderness after lovemaking. Oxytocin is also released at menstruation as the uterus contracts at this time of the cycle.

For so many women today, however, the lead up to their period is a source of great despair, pain, misery, temper outbursts, and tears. Yet even with these states of upset (which I want so much for you to be relieved of… please follow the advice in the solutions section as you do not need to put up with menstrual cycle challenges!) if you were to pause, you would notice that a calm state is available to you at this time.

In the West we have an epidemic of exhaustion. We push and push and push and don't allow ourselves enough downtime. There are very few women in the Western world who would not benefit enormously from more rest. For women, menstruation is the natural time for this and as a bonus during this time, an innate "natural calm" is on offer. Lifetsyle changes may need to be made however, to be able to soak up what is on offer at this time.

Slow down as you come into and during menstruation. Go to bed earlier. Apart from getting good quality rest, there is evidence that the extra dreaming time is good for easing PMS. Sleep is the all-round number one remedy, and it is free.

One of the strategies I suggest to women is to keep track of their menstrual period and reduce their commitments in the lead up to and during that time, particularly on day one of bleeding. Even if you have to go to work, do your best to not push yourself too hard that day. If what I've just written makes you roll your eyes and exclaim on the inside that I clearly have no idea what your life is like, take a breath. There are very few women in the Western world who don't have sixty million things on their plate. But every minute of every day you *choose* how to spend your time. Granted it may not be possible every single month to give yourself the gift of some downtime during menstruation, but do everything in your power to make this happen. Your body's innate wisdom guides you to do this. Women need to allow themselves to be guided by this more. Even just doing this, I've seen women have far more regular, less challenging menstruation. For girls or women with PCOS who may not menstruate, I suggest you schedule your downtime for the first night of the dark moon. Science and history teach us that the ovaries are stimulated by light. Historically, before electric light, women tended to ovulate on the full moon and bleed on the dark moon. I encourage all women to notice the moon as often as they can. If you have to go outside at night, don't just take the rubbish out or tend to the dog or run to your car, look up at the night sky and notice the moon. I encourage you to draw her silver light into your ovaries and imagine them being lit up. This is a particularly important exercise if you don't menstruate regularly. While you do this be sure to diaphragmatically breathe. Combined with attention to diet and herbs, this very feminine ritual can be incredibly beneficial to menstrual cycle health and calm.

Scientific research supports the need for more quiet time. A day of absolute solitude was found to be the best antidote for what were shown to be "overtaxed, overstuffed brains" and the ideal way to attain optimal brain performance. Another researcher claimed that "everyone in the study was chronically stimulated, socially and physically, and that we are probably operating at a stimulation level higher than that for which our species evolved." This scientist's remedy was to spend more time alone. Two other scientists also found that attentive listening to silence helps the human brain to focus, while what has been coined "conscious menstruation" by brilliant authors Jane Bennett and Alexandra Pope, has also been found to be a way to attain optimal brain performance. Slowing down and becoming more conscious are crucial to our well-being. If we ignore our need to "chillax" (as my best-friend's son says when he needs to chill out and relax all at once) or withdraw during menstruation, it may contribute to the development of some of the classic PMS symptoms such as disorientation, dreaminess, fogginess, feeling overwhelmed and irritable, as well as headaches and menstrual pain. However, if you can see your period as a time to turn down the volume, take a break, or perhaps just do less, the calm on offer will find you.

One of my clients who insists on going to the gym seven days a week decided to walk in nature instead on the days of her period to see if that helped. It has and she has now embraced this new ritual. Another lady got her closest friends together and asked them all to share their menstruation dates. They all plugged the dates into their phones and they make a point of getting in touch on the day their friends' periods are due to see if there is anything they can do to help out such as minding their children for a period of time that day. Gorgeous. Women are amazing.

Even if you lead a very high-pressured life with barely a moment to yourself, with only a simple change in attitude you can start to get a taste of the natural calm on offer to you at the time of your period. The next time it is day one of your cycle, the first day of bleeding, take a moment before you race (hopefully not!) into your day and notice how your body feels to you. Just acknowledge whatever you notice. Wonder to yourself that if you didn't have to work or worry about others today, what would I most love to do? Then, with curiosity rather than despair, drama or frustration, consider how you might give yourself twenty minutes of that on that day. When I've asked women this, the majority reply that they would love nothing better than simply curling up with a great book or a pile of magazines and not having to worry about anything or anyone. So ladies, please, examine your schedule and be ruthless about cutting out what is not essential on the first day of your period, even "fun" things like catching up with a friend for lunch. Notice how you might leak energy by getting caught up in drama, gossip, or having to listen to other people's problems. Do your best to excuse yourself from these situations as quickly as you can for this is the one day you need to receive. Do your best to eat well on this day too. At first simply become aware of this pattern in your month. The more aware of this cycle and this opportunity for calm you become, the more you will feel like you can make little changes that will open this stage up for you and the more effective you are also likely to be in your professional life. Renewal and rest are crucial to our health. You now need to allow it.

Menstruation and menopause are feminine and very natural processes. They offer incredible insight into a woman's general health as well as a window into her inner world of subconscious thoughts and beliefs. These thoughts and beliefs drive so much of what we do and how we feel. They can be a barometer guiding you to remember what you were born knowing… that you are the embodiment of loveliness.

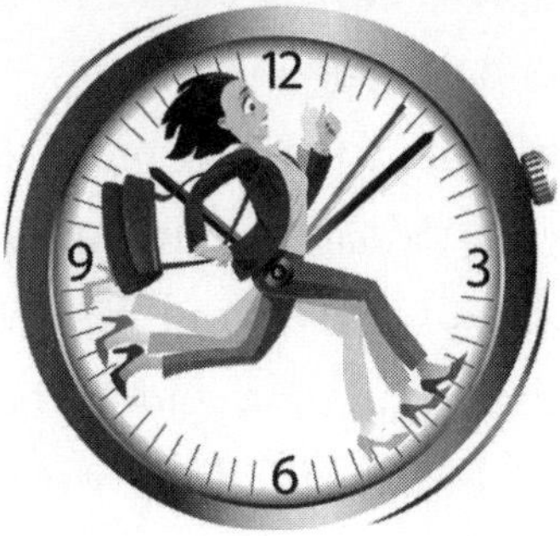

Chapter 3
Part 3
Your Thyroid and Your Thyroid Hormones: their role and impact on you in your rush

When it comes to feeling the rush, the thyroid gland is another part of the endocrine system that both contributes to and is affected by our environment and our perceptions. And again, the pituitary gland, in this case influenced by the hypothalamus, controls thyroid function. Understanding where any dysfunction may have come from and the mechanisms involved is crucial to improving your health, your body size and how you feel on a daily basis.

The thyroid gland is a little butterfly-shaped gland that sits in your throat area. It makes hormones that play an enormous role in your metabolic rate as well as temperature regulation and energy (i.e. not feeling fatigued). Every day of my working life, I meet people who exhibit virtually every symptom of an underactive thyroid, yet their blood test results demonstrate that everything is in the "normal" range. More on "normal" ranges later.

THE THYROID HORMONES

The production of thyroid hormones involves a cascade of signals, and glands other than the thyroid are also involved. This means that if you have a problem with thyroid hormone levels or with debilitating symptoms indicating something is awry with your thyroid function, then it is essential to get to the heart of the matter so treatment can be appropriately targeted.

The thyroid function cascade begins with the hypothalamus, a gland that makes a hormone that sends a signal to the pituitary gland, the tiny gland that sits at the base of your brain, which we've already seen produces hormones involved in menstruation. The pituitary in turn makes a hormone called thyroid stimulating hormone (TSH) that signals the thyroid to make one if its hormones known simply as T4 (thyroxine). T4 is found in the blood in two forms, namely T4 and free T4 (FT4). They are the same hormone, except one is "free" to enter tissues and the other is bound up and unable to enter tissues, which is where the work needs to be done. However, both T4 and FT4 are inactive hormones, and must be converted into the active thyroid hormone called T3 (triiodothyronine). It is T3 that drives your metabolic rate and capacity to burn body fat. The flow chart below illustrates the hormonal cascade.

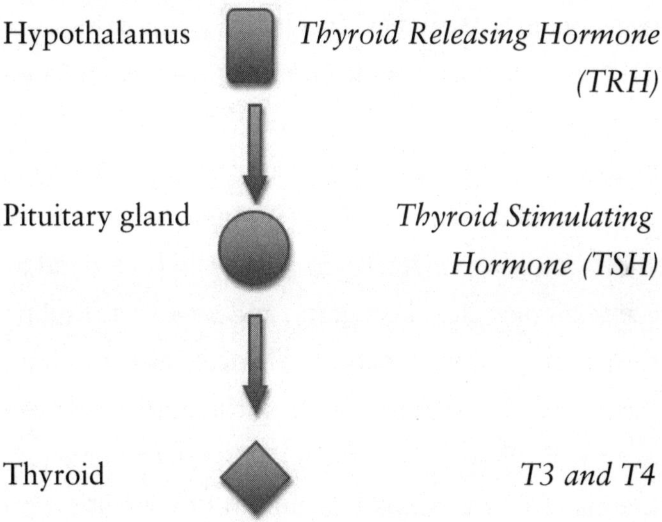

The Thyroid Hormone Cascade: *Signalling begins with the hypothalamus, followed by the pituitary which then in turn signals the thyroid gland to make its hormones.*

There are a number of nutrients essential to the production of optimal levels of thyroid hormones. Iodine and selenium are both vital minerals to this process of conversion that literally lights up your metabolic rate. Many people today get very little iodine and selenium in their diets as the majority of soils in the Western world do not contain these trace minerals and if the nutrients are not in the soil, they cannot be in the food that is grown in them.

The thyroid gland can become overactive, known as hyperthyroidism, or underactive, known as hypothyroidism, and it is the latter scenario that can lead to weight gain that can be difficult to shift until this issue is addressed. Some people swing between an underactive and an overactive situation. The thyroid gland is also susceptible to autoimmune diseases, meaning your immune system, which is supposed to defend you from infection, starts to see the thyroid gland as a foreign particle, like a germ, and attacks it, leading to a change in its function. This can lead to either the overactive picture (with autoimmune involvement this is known as Graves disease) or an underactive picture (known as Hashimoto's thyroiditis with autoimmune involvement). Infection, poor liver function, iodine, selenium, and iron deficiencies, as well as estrogen dominance or elevated cortisol, are all major factors that can initiate this process. Reread that list and think about what you have already learned from the earlier sections about stress hormones and sex hormones. It is important to work out the path that leads someone to altered thyroid function, for behind the "why" lies most of the answer.

HYPOTHYROIDISM: UNDERACTIVE THYROID GLAND FUNCTION

One of the first things that springs to mind with underactive thyroid people, is that they almost always tell me that coffee makes them happy and the first twenty minutes or so after they've had a coffee, is the only time they feel what they call "normal." A "thyroid person" will also usually tell me that chocolate helps them, and if they feel this way, it is potentially not just the caffeine content of the chocolate but it may also be due to the dopamine-enhancing actions of this food. Dopamine is a neurotransmitter that when in low supply can be involved in depression, while too much can drive addictive behaviours. For someone with poor thyroid function, chocolate may give them a little lift. Please don't necessarily assume that if you love chocolate that you are a "thyroid person"... many people simply love chocolate.

The classic symptoms of hypothyroidism are:

- Gradual weight increase over months for no apparent reason

- Often feeling cold, sometimes cold in your bones and like you can't get warm
- Tendency to constipation
- Tendency to depressed mood, forgetfulness, and a sense of being easily confused
- Hair loss or hair drier than previously
- Dry, brittle nails
- Menstrual problems
- Difficulty conceiving
- Beyond tired, you are fatigued
- Headaches

If a woman's thyroid gland is underactive, she is more likely to feel deeply fatigued and more depressed in her mood, rather than racy and anxious. However, I've met countless women who, from a mood and behaviour perspective, appear to bounce between these two extremes, so I felt it was important to explore both the under and overactive thyroid health pictures. And given that the thyroid is controlled by the pituitary, when the whole endocrine system is not able to work optimally due to your perception of pressure and a lack of "safety" in your world, the thyroid is a likely target for dysfunction.

Let's explore the roads to an underactive thyroid and where to begin to support your thyroid health.

INFECTION AND POOR LIVER DETOXIFICATION

A history (at any stage in life) of glandular fever (Epstein-Barr Virus, also know as mononucleosis), for example, can be a common road to hypothyroidism, as is liver overload, or a congested liver as I sometimes refer to it (and as was explained in the "Healthy Breasts" article in the sex hormone section). Treatment of both of these roads involves taking excellent care of the liver, and I encourage you to apply my liver-loving strategies outlined in the solutions chapter. Additionally, Astragalus is an excellent herb to use for a chronic infection background if an herbalist agrees this will meet your needs.

MINERAL DEFICIENCIES

Since hypothyroidism can be influenced by deficiencies in selenium, iodine, and iron—choose foods that are rich in these minerals. Eat brazil nuts daily for selenium. Use Celtic sea salt with iodine and/or cook with seaweeds such as Kombu for iodine. Good food sources of iron include beef, lamb, eggs, mussels, sardines, lentils, green leafy vegetables, and dates. There is a small amount of iron in many foods, so eating a varied diet is important. And remember that absorption is enhanced by vitamin C. If you do not eat animal foods, do not assume you are iron deficient. For some vegetarians, their body utilizes the iron from vegetable sources very efficiently. A blood test can be done for both iron and your iron storage (ferritin) levels.

The other option is to take a supplement that covers these nutrients. There are some excellent thyroid support capsules on the market so seek out one of these if it appeals. Regarding iron, it can be good to have a test before you supplement, as overloading on iron is not good. But if you are deficient it can be challenging and a very slow process to get your iron levels up without supplementation. So it is good to know your blood levels of this mineral. Many iron supplements are constipating, but most people find this doesn't happen with liquid iron supplements.

Here's some more on Iodine from a magazine article I wrote... just so you know how important this is!

> **Iodine**
>
> Iodine is a trace mineral so essential to our health that our body begins to shut down without it. Our thyroid gland loves iodine, and it cannot make thyroid hormones without it. Symptoms of an underactive thyroid include a deep tiredness and sluggish, heavy feeling; dry skin or hair; feelings of cold; a tendency to be constipated; puffy eyes; and a tendency to a depressed mood. Increasing dietary iodine intake can make a difference.

Thyroid hormones essentially determine our metabolic rate as adults and our growth as children. Iodine is also essential to the IQ of the developing brain *in utero* and, sadly, studies are now showing that some children in the Western world are suffering from such low iodine levels that their IQ is being detrimentally affected.

Why is this so?

Soil is a poor source of iodine, and if a nutrient is not in the soil it cannot be in our food. Where once foods made from whole grains, for example, were good sources in areas where the soil contained iodine in the first place, the depletion of the mineral content of our soils means this is no longer the case. New Zealand has volcanic soil, which has never contained any iodine. While the soil may not be a good source of iodine, the sea is somewhat better.

Food sources of iodine include all of the seaweeds, which you can add to soups, stews, casseroles, and salads to give them a subtle salty flavour while imparting all of the nutritional value of the minerals. A form of seaweed commonly eaten is nori, used frequently in sushi. Iodine is in small amounts in seafood, but even eating seafood every day will not provide you with adequate amounts of iodine.

Salt was first iodized in 1924; however, it tended to go out of "fashion" with the advent of rock salts and Celtic sea salt.

Although Celtic sea salt offers the additional benefits of a broad range of trace minerals, it lacks iodine unless it has been fortified. The only concern with conventional iodized salts is that most brands contain anti-caking agents that are not ideal for human health.

The impact of iodine therapy for the maintenance of healthy breast tissue has been widely reported, although it is rarely discussed. The ovaries also concentrate iodine, and studies have shown that a form of estrogen associated with breast cancer is produced by the ovaries in an iodine-deficient state. This has been shown to be reversible once iodine levels are optimal again.

Iodine is a difficult mineral to test for. Accurate tests require you to collect twenty-four hours of urine and, remarkably, not all countries offer this testing.

Adult females require 120 micrograms (µg), males 150 µg, of iodine per day to prevent deficiency. It is far more beneficial, however, to individualize doses. Often amounts between twelve and fifty milligrams (mg) are initially necessary to treat a deficient state, and this can be easily done with one to three drops of a good quality liquid iodine solution per day, available from some health food shops or through a compounding pharmacist. It is best to obtain specific advice to learn how to meet your individual needs.

~~~~~~~~~~~~~~~~
~~~~~~~~~~~~~~~~

ESTROGEN DOMINANCE

Too much estrogen can suppress thyroid function while optimal progesterone levels support its function. Apply the strategies for dealing with estrogen dominance outlined in the solutions chapter if you suspect that this is the basis for your challenge with your thyroid gland.

ELEVATED CORTISOL BROUGHT ON BY STRESS

Elevated cortisol as a result of stress decreases the levels of the active, fat burning thyroid hormone T3, which slows your metabolism. Added to this, high levels of cortisol urge your body to break down muscle to provide glucose for your brain, and reducing your muscle slows your metabolic rate as well. In the absence of stress, a healthy body converts FT4 into T3, but with elevated cortisol levels, the conversion of FT4 to T3 decreases.

Poor conversion of FT4 to active T3 also occurs if you restrict your food intake. Your body assumes that you must be starving, and therefore it must slow down the metabolic rate to preserve those precious fat stores. It may be frustrating, but your body's primary goal is always survival.

Elevated cortisol also inhibits the release of TSH from the pituitary and with less TSH, the body produces less FT4. Apply the strategies for high cortisol outlined in the solutions chapter if this scenario rings true for you. Poor thyroid function can also lead to elevated cholesterol, and once thyroid function has been treated, the cholesterol returns to normal.

THYROID MEDICATIONS

Typically today, if someone has been diagnosed with an underactive thyroid, they are prescribed thyroxine (T4). Some people feel brilliant on this medication and all of their hypothyroid symptoms disappear, including their weight gain. If this has not happened for you despite taking this medication, try a different approach. After years of taking thyroxine, it will not suddenly start to work if it hasn't yet.

There are numerous brands of thyroxine on the market. If you want to stick with conventional medicine, tell your general practitioner you feel lousy on your current medication (if you do) and that you would like to try a different drug. I have hundreds of clients who were happily taking one form of thyroxine and when the thyroid medication that is subsidised was changed to a different brand, all of their symptoms returned. Explore this even if your blood levels of TSH, FT4, and T3 are "normal," but you still have symptoms.

In my opinion, an excellent option to try when it comes to hypothyroidism is whole thyroid extract

(WTE). This is taken instead of any synthetic medication and, unlike the synthetics providing only one of the thyroid hormones, WTE provides all of the thyroid hormones. It is essential that you see your doctor about this and, if you so choose, be guided in the transition from a synthetic to the WTE, which is made by a compounding pharmacist.

If you have not been diagnosed with a thyroid illness, but you exhibit numerous symptoms, do not rely solely on your blood test results to determine if your thyroid is underactive. Work with a health professional who will treat the symptoms, not the blood, and who will monitor both your symptoms and the blood work as you explore treatments. I learned this in a powerful way with a client whose story melts my heart.

THYROID ANTIBODIES

The importance of testing thyroid antibodies is best demonstrated with this story. A precious lady arrived at my practice for assistance with her health, and when I asked how I could help, she burst into tears and said she knows she has had an underactive thyroid for about thirty years. Patricia's blood tests always come back within the normal range, and she said no one would treat her. She had gained over 100 kilos (220 pounds) over thirty years, and it all began when her dear mother passed away. Patricia said she had eaten poorly for about three to four months after her mom's death, and put on weight, but her grief gradually eased and, as it did, she started to eat better again, as she always had. But nothing changed. Her size kept increasing. So then she didn't just eat well, she signed up for a gym membership, and she started to eat even better. When I saw her, Patricia was unable to exercise due to knee pain from carrying so much weight (her description and she thought she was "about 180 kilograms" (400 pounds), but she still ate in a way that did not warrant her size.

Of course Patricia had a huge amount of unresolved grief (for which she said doctors [with the best of intentions] kept offering her antidepressants that she always declined because she felt it was her thyroid), and yes there had been times when she hadn't eaten very well. But she had also had plenty of months and years of making extraordinary efforts for no reward.

Given that Patricia ticked every box when it came to symptoms of an underactive thyroid, I decided to request fresh blood tests and include thyroid antibodies, specifically anti-thyroid peroxidase and anti-thyroglobulin. Having been taught at university that it was highly unlikely for thyroid antibodies to be elevated and an issue if thyroid hormone levels were in the normal range, I could understand why Patricia's autoantibodies had not been tested—but from a symptoms perspective I could not.

To cut a very long story short, despite her latest thyroid hormones levels being in the "normal" range, but skewed one way (discussed below), Patricia's antibodies were the highest I have ever seen. To put this in context, the "normal" range for both of these antibodies tests in this national laboratory is less than fifty (<50). Patricia's anti-thyroid peroxidase and anti-thyroglobulin were both >6500—off the scale and through the roof. When I phoned to tell her, she was at first thrilled that all along there had been a reason for how lousy she had felt. She told me later that anger then surfaced for a life she felt she'd missed out on because this was not picked up. She had remained very shy, which she blamed on her size, and on reflection was very sad that she had not met a partner with whom to share her life. She decided to seek out the most natural approach she could for her very underactive thyroid, and after considerable weight fell off her over the first three months, she booked her first overseas holiday. There is always a why. You just have to find it.

HYPERTHYROIDISM: OVERACTIVE THYROID GLAND FUNCTION

Common signs and symptoms of an overactive thyroid include:

- Heart palpitations
- Heat intolerance or easily overheating (this can also indicate liver congestion)
- Nervousness
- Insomnia
- Breathlessness
- Increased bowel movements
- Light or absent menstrual periods
- Fatigue but more wired than tired
- Fast heart rate
- Trembling hands
- Weight loss (although not always as appetite increases with hyperthyroidism and some people eat enough to cover the increase in metabolism)
- Muscle weakness
- Warm, moist skin
- Hair loss
- Staring gaze
- Bulging eyes

Thyroid hormones have a direct effect on most organs, including the heart, which beats faster and harder under the influence of thyroid hormones. Essentially, all cells in the body will respond to increases in thyroid hormone levels with an increase in the rate at which they conduct their business.

When it comes to an overactive thyroid, whether there is autoimmune involvement (Graves disease) or not, a frantic pace of life has been involved with every single case I have worked with. In my experience, stress, specifically the pace of life and what each woman has demanded of her body, is the major factor in the development of hyperthyroidism. More than any other group, they have sacrificed sleep and they have juggled more in their lives to date than most people could juggle in a lifetime. As I like to say to one of my favourite rushing friends, "it is as if you run a small country" with all that she handles. And there is usually a part of them that actually quite enjoys life this way. They are often at a bit of a loss as to why their body has gone and done this to them (presented with elevated anti-thyroid antibodies along with elevated thyroid hormone function tests). Yet their body has sent them a powerful message that the way in which they were living was not serving their health or perhaps even their destiny and what life had in store for them. I believe that your body does its best to wake you up to pay attention to what *really* needs your attention, every day. I've seen some overactive thyroid conditions return to normal with this acknowledgement and the subsequent lifestyle change that must go with it.

All of the women I've worked with who have successfully returned their thyroid function to normal (from being overactive), and had a complete remission of their symptoms, have literally changed their life. They usually change their jobs and, if that is not possible, they completely change their approach and attitude to that work and their life. It has been inspiring to witness in my clients. Louise Hay suggests there is a feeling of "rage at being left out," and she encourages people to affirm "I am the centre of my life, and I approve of myself and all that I see."

It is virtually impossible to slow down and approach life from a calm, centred space when your body is getting the message that it needs to speed everything up. So the physical aspect of this condition most certainly needs to be sorted out. It can be very difficult to take part in a meditation class when your heart feels like it is about to jump out of your chest. However, I want to encourage you to also get to the real reason of why you may have run your life at such an intense pace in the first place. The whys are explored in the emotions chapter.

BLOOD TESTS AND "NORMAL" RANGES

The concept of a normal range is necessary as cutoff

points help indicate when something may be abnormal. I have great concerns, however, when we base the future of a person's health on blood tests alone.

According to Dr. Karen Coates, an insightful and pioneering general practitioner and coauthor of *Embracing The Warrior: An Essential Guide for Women*, the normal range for some blood tests is calculated periodically by each pathology laboratory to ensure that the reference range printed on the test results is "accurate." On the morning of this day, the first one hundred blood samples received are tested for their (in this case) TSH levels in order to determine the reference range. Or it might be iron levels for example. But! Why do people usually have blood tests? Because they are feeling particularly spritely that day? No! Most often, the precise opposite is true! Yet it seems we base our "normal" ranges on these figures. Furthermore, it is also important to understand how the "average" amount of a particular nutrient or hormone is calculated. Mathematically, the top reference point is calculated to be "two standard deviations" above the average, while the bottom figure is "two standard deviations" below the average. The arbitrary rules of this method dictate that 95 percent of the one hundred blood samples taken must fall into the "normal" range. The statistical definition of standard deviations insists that only four or five results may fall outside this reference range, two samples below and two above.

The two points I want to make are: first, the reference ranges for some blood parameters are getting broader. The normal range for TSH when I wrote the first draft of my previous book *Accidentally Overweight* was 0.4 to 4.0. By the time the book went to publication four months later, the normal range had been expanded to 0.3 to 5.0. As mentioned later, people at either end of this blood range will look and feel completely different and they will more than likely exhibit thyroid symptoms. If they are symptom free, no problem, their body is not trying to draw their attention to the thyroid gland. However, my concern is this: if we base treatment on the blood work alone and leave people to live with their symptoms with their result skewed to one end of the normal range, we are risking, not optimizing, their health. This brings me to my next point, which is that you can see from the start that this process is flawed, given it is done on individuals who are potentially unwell. It is more challenging to create optimal health, prevent disease, and maximize quality of life for people when they are being guided with their blood tests to fall into a potentially unhealthy normal range.

I urge you to get copies of your own blood tests and look for results being skewed to one end of the normal range. Let me explain.

The normal range for TSH where I live is currently 0.4 to 4.0 (it switched back to this range). Although those numbers may seem small, someone with a TSH of 0.4 feels and looks completely different from someone with a TSH of 4. Additionally, if your results are not actually outside the normal range, you will usually be told (well-meaningly) that there is no problem with your thyroid. A common picture I see is a TSH of 2.5 or greater (made by the pituitary) screaming out to the thyroid gland to make FT4. FT4 normal levels are between ten and twenty and usually, for someone with symptoms of hypothyroidism, their FT4 will be eleven. This person feels exhausted in their bones, has trouble naturally using their bowels daily, has dry skin, very low motivation, a tendency to a depressed mood, brain fog, and their clothes are gradually getting tighter. Their thyroid needs support.

In this case, I always start with iodine and selenium and sometimes iron, along with adrenal support, a grain-free diet, and a big chat about their beliefs and what their perception is of what life is like for them.

Louise Hay, the brilliant metaphysical medicine pioneer, teaches that thyroid problems represent feelings and beliefs around humiliation and feeling like you never get to do what you want to do (how many mothers—in particular—does that describe?!?). Louise Hay suggests someone with thyroid problems unconsciously asks, "When is it going to be my turn?" She suggests you develop a new thought pattern of "I move beyond old limitations and now allow myself to express freely and creatively." Underneath diagnosed hypothyroidism, Louise Hay suggests, are feelings of hopelessness, a feeling of being stifled, and a sense of giving up. She suggests you develop a new thought pattern of "I create a new life with new rules that totally support me."

I include this information to offer you a whole picture of your thyroid health, from the conventional function of hormones and glands and blood tests; through the nutritional supports that are essential, including iodine and selenium; to the metaphysical. Somewhere among these three approaches lies your answer, not necessarily in one or the other. I urge you to explore all three.

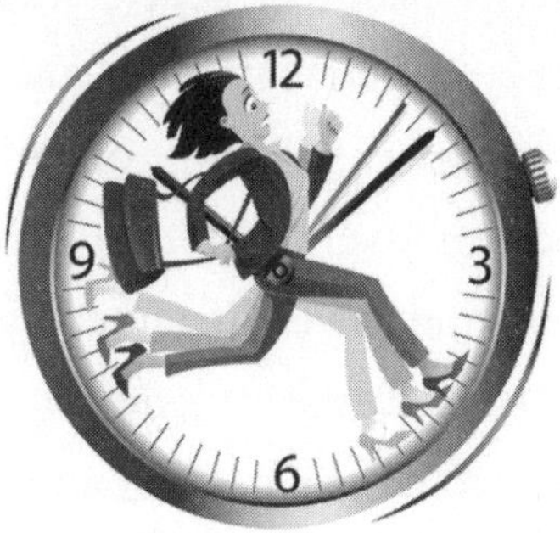

Chapter 3 Part 4

The Pituitary Gland: the vital role of the master gland in every aspect of women's health

Part of what I always aim to do for people, is get to the heart of their health matter. This usually involves exploring what is happening for them physically and emotionally. There are numerous body systems intricately involved in our physical and emotional health, how we look, how we feel, and how we behave. And as you have just read, as well as the nervous system, the endocrine system holds the key to so much about how we feel. The master control centre for our hormonal systems is the pituitary gland, a gland that is often overlooked when exploring women's health unless symptoms distinctively point to a problem in this area. Yet creating an environment inside the body that allows the pituitary gland to work optimally can be the key to nullifying the panic as well as regulating all of the other endocrine glands including the adrenals, the ovaries, and the thyroid.

WHAT DOES THE PITUITARY GLAND CONTROL?

The pituitary gland is a pea-sized gland located at the base of the skull between the optic nerves, and its main task is to secrete hormones. The reason the pituitary is sometimes referred to as the "master gland" is that it controls hormone functions such as our temperature, thyroid activity, growth during childhood, urine production, and ovulation. In effect the gland functions as our thermostat that controls all other glands that are responsible for hormone secretion. The gland is a critical part of our ability to respond to the environment most often without our knowledge. It is the link between our nervous system and our endocrine systems. The chart shows the location of the pituitary gland, housed in the brain about level with the bridge of your nose, and the glands it affects.

The Pituitary and Its Target Glands

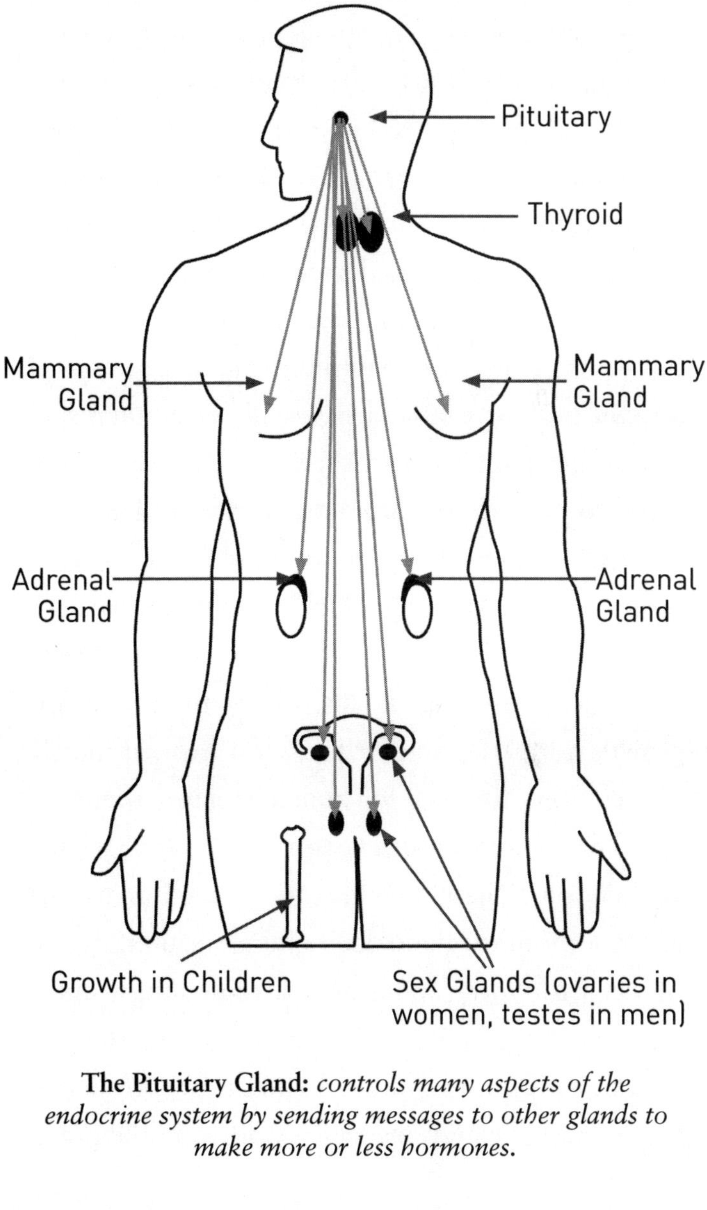

The Pituitary Gland: *controls many aspects of the endocrine system by sending messages to other glands to make more or less hormones.*

The pituitary gland actually functions as two separate compartments: an anterior (front) portion and the posterior (back) portion. The anterior gland is made up of a separate collection of individual cells that act as individual factories (correctly termed "functional units") that are dedicated to produce a specific regulatory hormone messenger or factor. These factors are secreted in response to the outside environment and the internal bodily responses to this environment. These pituitary factors then travel into the bloodstream and eventually reach their specific target gland. There they stimulate the target gland to produce the appropriate type and amount of hormone so the body can respond to the environment correctly. Isn't that alone absolutely amazing?

There are "factories" for a number of specific hormones including a cortisol factory, one for growth hormone, one for prolactin (related mostly to lactation), another for gonadotropin (stimulates the gonads), and another factory for thyroid-related stimulation. These five factories function as the anterior pituitary gland neuroendocrine unit. Again, no need to worry about any of these long-winded scientific names... I simply want you to see that the pituitary plays the role of the master controller of the endocrine glands we have explored in the previous sections.

The posterior part of the pituitary stores and secretes hormones made by the hypothalamus. Both sections of the pituitary are directly connected to, and controlled by, the hypothalamus, a section of the brain controlling the basic survival processes of hunger, thirst, sexual reproduction, and self-defence. A stem containing both neurons (the nervous system) and small blood vessels (to transport the hormones of the endocrine system) connects the pituitary gland with the hypothalamus. Therefore, the hypothalamus communicates with the pituitary in two ways: by nerve impulses and by chemical messengers (hormones). The anterior pituitary receives instructions from the hypothalamus in the form of releasing hormones. These chemical messengers produced by the hypothalamus then travel through the blood. A special network of vessels directs this blood through the anterior pituitary. In contrast, the posterior pituitary receives its messages through neural tissue and is controlled by nerve impulses.

If any one of the factories in the anterior part of the pituitary become excited and start to overproduce their respective hormonal factor, the net result is excess production of the final hormone product. For example, if the cortisol cells, called corticotrophs, lose their ability to respond to the normal stimuli from the environment and from the hypothalamus and develop their own independent, uncontrolled autonomous secretion, they will produce more cortisol than the body requires. In return the adrenal glands will be overstimulated and secrete unregulated and unneeded stress chemicals, called "catecholamines." The net result is excess production of these important chemicals that can signal fat storage, affect blood pressure (usually elevate it) and drive the heart rate higher, among other things. This can cause the body and internal organs to be stressed when there is no need. Unfortunately, the consequences of overdriving the internal organs of the body can take a toll on your health and, eventually, be life threatening. In extreme cases, the cells that overproduce their respective hormones can clump together within a given area of the pituitary gland creating a true factory of overproduction which would be diagnosed as a pituitary tumour. Not all pituitary tumours are cancerous, however all tumours need medical attention due to the hormonal dysregulation they promote.

WHAT HORMONES DOES THE PITUITARY MAKE?

The pituitary gland makes six hormones from the front part of the gland and two from the back. The front part makes:

- Thyroid Stimulating Hormone (TSH)

    - Signals the thyroid gland to make thyroid hormones

- Lutenizing Hormone (LH)
    - Signals the ovaries
- Follicle Stimulating Hormone (FSH)
    - Signals the ovaries
- Prolactin
    - Stimulates breast development and breast milk production
- Growth hormone
    - For the growth of all tissues in the body
- Adrenocorticotrophic hormone (ACTH)
    - Signals to the adrenals to make cortisone (which is converted into cortisol)

The back part makes:

- Antidiuretic hormone (ADH)
    - Controls how much urine is passed
- Oxytocin
    - Asks the uterus to contract at appropriate times in life (e.g. during childbirth and orgasm)

There are other endocrine glands in the body that do not need the pituitary gland to give them messages to produce their hormones. These glands include the parathyroids for calcium regulation and the pancreas for insulin production. They are controlled through other mechanisms.

To give you an example of how one of these pituitary hormones works, let's look at ACTH, whose job it is to direct the adrenal glands, whose function is essential to life. The hypothalamus produces an ACTH-releasing factor that stimulates ACTH secretion from the pituitary into the bloodstream. Specifically programmed receptors on the adrenal glands pick up the ACTH and these receptors start sending signals to the centre of the cells (known as the cell nucleus) to start producing and secreting adrenal hormones. These hormones are then released into the circulatory system and their presence is communicated to the brain. The broad (family) names for some of these hormones include the glucocorticoids (such as cortisol), which influence the metabolism of the body, the mineralocorticoids (such as aldosterone) which are involved in regulating the amount of water in the body and hence blood pressure; and progesterone, which as you know is a hormone crucial to reproduction as it prepares the uterus for the reception and preparation of a fertilized egg (ovum).

Like so many other hormones, ACTH is secreted in a circadian pattern over a twenty-four-hour period. Each individual has their own internal circadian rhythm which determines how much sleep that person needs, when they are most alert, and when they prefer to eat. Disruptions of this rhythm can affect biological functions, moods, as well as intellectual ability. For example, jet lag after a flight across a multitude of time zones is probably the result of a disruption of the circadian rhythm.

For most people, ACTH is at its highest blood level in the early morning and, with its action on the adrenals and the subsequent hormones that are produced, it influences whether you bound or crawl out of bed, and because the adrenals are the place from which we make our stress hormones, it seems, over time, that if the stress goes on for too long, they become less able to adapt to our surroundings. In other words, they are getting the message that they need to make stress hormones when you may, in fact, be safe.

OBVIOUS SYMPTOMS OF PITUITARY PROBLEMS

When there is significant dysfunction with the pituitary gland, the following symptoms are common:

- Headaches
- Visual disturbances

- Fatigue and lethargy
- Inability to cope
- Unexpected abnormal growth
- Sleep disturbance
- Nipple discharge
- Impotence (men)
- Absence or disturbance of the menstrual cycle
- Skin and hair changes

Not everyone will experience all of these symptoms at all or at once. These signs and symptoms may occur because the target organ is not working effectively, it may not be the "fault" of the pituitary gland itself. There are tests an endocrinologist can run to determine what precisely is going on. When there is a diagnosed pituitary condition, it will usually be necessary for an endocrinologist to prescribe the hormones to be replaced.

SUBOPTIMAL PITUITARY FUNCTION (NO DISEASE)

I have seen countless women display symptoms that involve all or most of the organs the pituitary governs without them having a full-blown pituitary condition. I call this suboptimal pituitary function.

These women will display symptoms involving the adrenal glands (related to stress hormones), often the reproductive system (e.g. PMS, PCOS, endometriosis, debilitating menopause), and sometimes the thyroid. If these women read information on the Internet they will tell me they can't work out if their problem is their adrenals, their sex hormones, or their thyroid as they relate to the symptoms (described in each previous section in this endocrine chapter) of dysfunction for each gland. They are usually tired but wired and they rarely sleep well. Their moods change easily and unpredictably and they are often impatient with the people they love the most in this world. And then berate themselves for being this way… hardly a winning formula for a happy life. If it is not clear to me based on the symptoms, I will test the stress hormones, the sex hormones, and thyroid function to get a clearer picture. And what has become apparent to me, is that for so many women today, all three of these systems are affected and not only do each of the affected glands need support, the pituitary does too.

I believe that this is the result of subconscious fear which is at the heart of why we rush. As I will explore in the emotions section, this fear can be due to real threat or perceived "threat." I meet countless women who tell me that they are in love. And they are! And yet they are also in fear... fear that they will not do a good enough job, fear that they are not there enough for their children, fear their intimate relationship will end unless they are a certain way, fear that they will go broke, fear that they will get yelled at... and so they do all in their power to avoid ever having to feel that they are not enough (because it instinctively triggers the switch that they won't be loved... remember the Introduction?). To prevent their fears from becoming realities, they go into overdrive, which, for some women, appears to take its toll on the pituitary gland and the glands it controls.

CONTROL

Here's the "weirdo medicine" aspect of how I consider health conditions... if the pituitary gland is the control centre for the human body, then it seems logical to conclude that this gland will be particularly effected in women who describe themselves as "control freaks," women who have forgotten how to trust the unfolding of life, that it is all part of a bigger picture that we can't often see or understand, and they've forgotten to be present in every moment.

I was reminded recently of the joy we can, as adults, so easily miss. I was sitting on a park bench watching people from all walks of life enjoy the sun and the outdoors. A mother threw a ball to her two sons (ages eight and ten), one of whom had a developmental delay. He didn't catch the ball every time she threw it to him while her other son did. When the developmentally typical boy caught the ball, he had no change of expression on his face, nor in his manner, and he simply threw the ball back to his mother. The boy with the developmental delay, however, celebrated every time he caught it! The delight and the excitement every time he caught the ball was as amped up as the first time he caught it, and he literally jumped with joy every time before he threw it back to his mother. Catching the ball had become routine to the younger, developmentally typical child, and he had lost his connection of glee to his ability, while the developmentally delayed child was truly living in the moment and outwardly demonstrating how thrilled he was with his achievement every time it happened.

How many of your own skills do you take for granted and no longer notice? Do you still pause at the feeling of human contact, someone else's skin on yours? Or the feeling of your pet's fur under your fingertips? Do you pause and breathe and tune in to how this feels? It is ultimately feminine to feel. The first time you felt these things, it would have felt like magic to you. Pause long enough in each moment to experience the magic. It is on offer 24/7. Only when we take our life for granted and tune out, and when we rush, we go momentarily blind. It is time to live your life in the light again and allow your pituitary gland to flourish.

AM I "SAFE"?

The typical health picture I am witnessing in more and more women is this... The hypothalamus asks the question "am I safe?" 24/7. It has always done this. In doing so, it is assessing your physical environment... is it too hot, too cold... and also emotionally. Trouble is, you have beliefs that you don't even know you have. You create meanings from the looks on people's faces and the things they say, based on what you experienced as a child whether you realize this or not. You think the world is how the world is, not how it really is. You tell yourself stories constantly about who you are and who and what you have to be. And, if based on the meanings you have set up in your nervous system, your hypothalamus perceives that you are not safe (from being yelled at or criticized, for example) then it, without you knowing, sends a message to the pituitary gland which fires off the sympathetic nervous system and all of the necessary hormones so you are ready to fight or flee.

That means the adrenals make adrenalin and/or

cortisol and most often both. Your adrenal production of progesterone is therefore decreased meaning you lose this vital antianxiety agent, and estrogen becomes dominant which makes you fleshy, puffy, and kind of crazy. This means your thyroid gets a signal to either amp up or decrease its hormone production, and your blood glucose is not astutely regulated which can lead you to feel like you want to eat your arm off. All of the above make it harder and harder to sleep well, further setting you up, biochemically, to rush. The "not feeling safe" feeds the cycle. And the chemistry the cycle elicits keeps it going.

But when I spell it out like that, you can see where you may need to start... with your own mind. Of course I will offer you solutions for the various hormonal pictures I've just described in the coming chapters—that is a huge part of what I do and why people's health improves—and of course I will encourage you to step up and do all you can to give your body the opportunity it is screaming out for to balance your sex hormones and stop churning out stress hormones, and reinvigorate your thyroid. There is much you can do to assist your body to do this. Yet at the same time, if I don't strongly urge you to literally get to the heart of your matter, and see *why* you rush, why you don't feel "safe," it is like trying to stop a bath from overflowing by easing the plug out of the hole to allow a small amount of water to escape. Exploring the emotional side of your health allows you to turn off the tap. Real food fosters that exploration, that enquiry. One of my key messages is this: It is very difficult to be kind, compassionate, and patient with others when you are filling yourself with stimulants and food that contains very little nutritional value. Choose real food that nourishes you, and watch your physical as well as your emotional health shine.

So all I want for you right now at this stage in the book, it to recognize the body systems that may need support. Don't worry about how you are going to do that right now. Just recognize, with immense compassion for yourself, that it is what it is. And the power to change your health is in your hands. And I achingly want to help you.

THE INTENSE STRESS OF NATURAL DISASTERS

There have tragically been many disasters in the world of late, both natural (such as earthquakes) and domestic (such as violence), and when I talk about stress I certainly do not want to make small of anything any of us may have been through. A natural disaster promotes the fight or flight response for a very good reason... to help you get out of danger and save your life. I know for many thousands of women I have met who have been through these events that the stress internally continues long after the events themselves may have passed. I admire your courage and resilience. And along with some additional understanding of the stress response, I offer you an article I wrote for a women's magazine after the earthquakes in Christchurch, New Zealand. Although some of the information you will have read in the adrenal and stress hormones section, I left the article intact to reiterate the power of both human biochemistry and human hearts! And I also offer you this statement: The impact and meaning of a catastrophe are not in the event itself. The ability to tolerate it is a function not of what has occurred but of our relationship to ourselves and our own minds. In the simplicity of that realisation is freedom.

The Stress Response

Given all that has happened in our beautiful country recently, exploring ways we can support our health physically, mentally, and emotionally in times of stress is of more importance than ever. Firstly let's examine what is going on inside the body in the aftermath of trauma and also the ongoing stress of what may be a deep worry about the future, experienced by many New Zealanders at this time.

Humans have an extraordinary resilience, both mentally and physically, and the body has an innate capacity to heal. Remember that! We really are amazing. However, to assist that process, there is much we can do to support our body's stress response. Here, I describe the physicality of the stress response not so you worry more but so that if your body, health, or mind-set start to change, you can rest assured that it is a natural process and that your body has an extraordinary capacity to heal.

Stage 1

Adrenalin is our acute stress hormone, the one that makes our heart race. It can make us shake, drive our thoughts to race, and makes us jump when we are startled. It also stops our digestive system working optimally as adrenalin wants you to stay focused on whatever is threatening your life. Adrenalin puts us on "red alert" meaning that we are geared to fight or flee. Initially, when we get a shock, this is the survival response of the body designed to get us out of danger.

This is the primary stress hormone that will have been made by anyone involved in, or directly affected by, the recent earthquakes. Some people get biochemically stuck in this state because the fear of another earthquake or concerns for family continues psychologically. Sleep can then be affected since your body's perception is that your life is in danger. If you do sleep deeply, your body is concerned you won't be ready to fight or flee. The best tactic on the planet to calm yourself from this state is to change your focus to something for which you are grateful (and I don't say that flippantly) and shift your breathing back into a pattern that makes your belly move in and out with each breath, rather than your chest. Nothing communicates to your nervous system that you are safe better than diaphragmatic breathing.

There are also herbs you can take that can assist and these include Withania, Passionflower, and Zizyphus. Keeping hydrated is also essential as is additional vitamin B (found in whole grains), vitamin C (found in many fruits and capsicum) and magnesium (found in green leafy vegetables and nuts).

Stage 2

After the initial shock, the second stage of stress is typically initiated. This involves the production of a different stress hormone called cortisol, which historically humans only produced in excess during floods, famines, or wars; all times when food was scarce. As a result of this, cortisol often makes you eat too much food, because when food abounds, your cortisol-fuelled body thinks you are so lucky to have found a whole packet of rice crackers!

Sleep is effected in this state too, however, this poor sleep generally means you fall asleep OK but you wake between 2:00am and 3:00am, when cortisol naturally rises. Cortisol initially does wonderful things for the body in this state of stress, as it is a powerful anti-inflammatory. We need the anti-inflammatory action to protect us from the metabolic inflammation adrenalin can cause. The problem for our health is when the stress goes on too long for the body to handle (which is different for everyone) as then cortisol starts to break down your muscles, suppress your immune system, and make your desire for sweet food almost uncontrollable. Excellent ways to support yourself through a period of elevated cortisol include doing your breathing exercises daily, using herbs such as Siberian ginseng, Rhodiola, Licorice, or Withania, and filling your diet with as many fresh foods as you can.

Stage 3

The next biochemical stage of stress that can occur, especially if the stress has been prolonged, may involve cortisol falling low. If you have had a high level of cortisol output for many, many years, your adrenal glands may not be able to stand the tension and so they crash. In general terms, you "burnout." In more recent times, this has become known as adrenal fatigue, because the major symptom now is an unrelenting, deep fatigue.

Cortisol is supposed to be high in the morning, and ideal amounts help you bounce out of bed. It plays a role in how vital you feel and helps the body combat any inflammatory processes that want to kick in. Stiffness is a key symptom of adrenal fatigue. For those with chronic stress, morning cortisol levels tend to be low and it can be very difficult to get out of bed with such low levels. By mid-afternoon, it will be at an all-time low, and you feel you need something sweet, something containing caffeine, or a nap to get you through your afternoon. For an adrenally fatigued person, cortisol is nice and low in the evenings, but if you don't go to bed before 10:00pm, you will typically get a second wind, and it will be much harder for you to fall asleep if you're still up at midnight. The fatigue you feel with this biochemical picture may make exercise the least appealing thing on the planet to you. You actually feel worse after exercise when you are adrenally fatigued, whereas exercise typically energises. For people with deep, deep fatigue, I almost always use the following herbal tonic that contains:

- Panex ginseng
- Licorice
- Dandelion leaves
- Astragalus

- One other herb depending on what else is going for the individual (a liver herb or a reproductive herb are typical)

I will also sometimes use a range of supplements from the United States, created by Dr James Wilson, specifically for adrenal fatigue. I have had countless clients take this range of supplements for three months and have their energy and vitality return to great levels.

Humans were never designed to sustain long-term stress, and our individual bodies cope with it in different ways. For some, adrenalin remains the dominant stress hormone all of their life, while others may flip over into a more cortisol-dominant stress response. If the stress response doesn't truly switch off, there is the potential that the adrenals will eventually crash, and cortisol output is no longer optimum or elevated. It is negligible. At its extreme, this condition is called Addison's disease, yet if a person has an extremely low cortisol level but that level still falls just inside the "normal" range, that person will be told that they are fine. They feel lousy, yet all of the tests they have always come back "normal." They feel anything but normal, and people who know and love them will often comment that they are a shell of their former selves.

Long-term, cortisol can also be rather sinister in that it can interfere with your steroid (sex) hormone metabolism, your sleep patterns via its interference with melatonin, and also your mood via serotonin.

Diet

Although I often recommend supplements of herbs and/or nutrients during times of stress, never underestimate the healing and restorative power of food the way it comes in nature. Taking supplements is not a reason to eat a poor quality, low nutrient diet. I simply recommend supplements where appropriate and especially to assist in the restoration of health.

Finally, human kindness goes such a long way towards healing and we have been privileged to witness such extraordinary acts. The courage of this nation is spectacular.

~~~~~~~~~~~~~~~~~~~
~~~~~~~~~~~~~~~~~~~

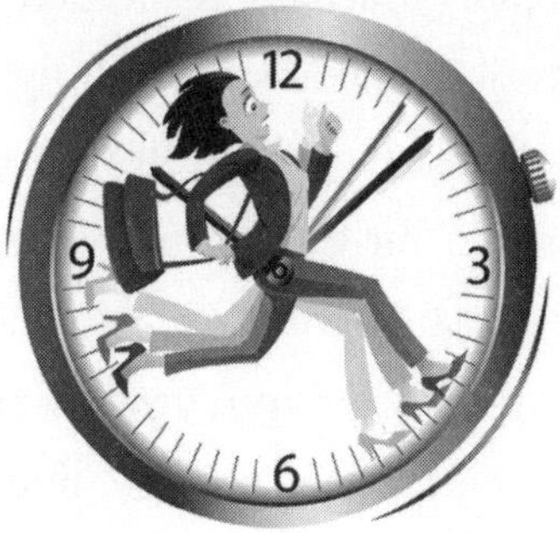

Chapter 4

The Digestive System: the impact of your rush on digestion

It never ceases to amaze me how magnificent and clever our bodies are, and I am astounded by how many processes go on inside our bodies without us having to give them any thought. Digestion is one of those processes. The nourishment provided to our bodies as a result of good digestion is an extraordinary gift without which we would not survive. Digestion is the process through which we extract all of the goodness out of our food. Digestion is intricate and complex but still relatively robust, and it is intimately connected to how you feel and function every single day, from the energy you have to the fat you burn, from the texture and appearance of your skin to whether you have a bloated tummy or not. In fact, digestion impacts everything, right down to your mood. It is responsible for so much that goes on inside us. If your digestion gives you grief, if you are bloated most evenings, if you have intermittent diarrhoea and constipation, or if you get reflux—you can reach a point where you feel like it is how life is always going to be. It must just be how you are. Perhaps you believe it's "in your family." Well, hear this: bowel challenges do not have to be your reality.

Unfortunately for more than 70 percent of women in the Western world, a condition called irritable bowel syndrome (IBS) has become the bane of their life. They do not have a bowel disease but rather a functional disorder of the digestive system, the symptoms of which can range from mild to debilitating. The main symptoms include diarrhoea, constipation and/or intermittent bouts of both, excessive flatulence, mucous in the stools, and a bloated tummy. I know I see a biased group of the population in my practice, but nine out of every ten women who see me about their health say yes when I ask them if they have a bloated stomach. Food is not supposed to bloat you, ladies.

Before I thoroughly explain IBS and offer you specific advice about what to do about it, it is crucial that you first understand how your digestive system works, as you may identify aspects of what you are experiencing with your tummy along the way. It is also important that you understand more about your digestive system, as it can be a challenge to sort your stress hormone production, for example, if your digestion is constantly giving you grief. The gut is essentially like a second brain in your body. Did you know that 80 percent of the body's total serotonin is in the gut? And as serotonin is our primary happy, calm, content hormone, gut dysfunction can enormously affect your mood.

Some of the information in this section may make you giggle… it can be a challenge to find the right words to describe bowel movements! And some of the advice may at first seem obvious and too simple to make much of a difference. And although I explored some of this in my book *Accidentally Overweight* I wanted to go into even more detail here, as the impact of rushing, stress, and urgency, whether you display it in your behaviour or hold it all in, on your digestion can be so powerful. So reflect on your own eating habits and digestive system functions as you read on, and be ready to resolve any frustrations you have with your digestive system.

HOW THE DIGESTIVE SYSTEM WORKS

Digestion is the process of breaking food down into smaller and smaller components; for example, proteins are broken down into amino acids so that we can absorb them and use them for energy and nourishment. This ongoing cascade of events sustains our life and it is truly amazing.

The digestive system is made up of a digestive tract—a big long tube (imagine it looking like a hose)—and numerous ancillary organs, including the liver, gall bladder, and pancreas. The tube begins at your mouth, where the digestion process begins with chewing. Food then moves down the esophagus, through a valve, and into your stomach. It then travels through another valve at the bottom end of the stomach and into the small intestine, through the small intestine and ileocaecal valve into the large intestine, and finally any waste is excreted out the other end. When this process works well, you look and feel fantastic. If it is in any way impaired, however, the opposite can be true, and resolving your symptoms can literally change your life.

CHEW YOUR FOOD

Food enters the mouth and moves down the esophagus into the stomach. But what do we do to our food before it reaches the stomach? We chew it or, in some cases, we inhale it! For obvious reasons you can't chew your food anymore once it has left your mouth. Yet so many people eat as though their esophagus is lined with teeth. Many of us are in such a hurry over our meals or simply with life in general, or perhaps we're so excited by the food's flavour that we might only chew each mouthful four times, if we're lucky. It's often a case of chew, chew, chew, chew mmm mmm yum, next forkful in, chew, chew, oh gosh my mouth is so full, better swallow some food… So we swallow some partially chewed food—and some food that hasn't been chewed at all—and we do this day in, day out, year after year. Often we aren't even aware that we do so. And somehow we expect our stomach to cope.

In the end, of course, your stomach gets to a point where it doesn't like the rushing rules by which you are playing. It has no time to prepare itself for the influx of food with the production of stomach acid and digestive enzymes. And given that all of the hormones (for example, adrenalin) and the messages being communicated by your nervous system (sympathetic nervous system activation) are telling your body that your life is in danger, you have no resources available to digest food. Your body believes it needs to fight or run rather than rest and digest.

So, slow down and chew your food well. If you find this challenging and are a food inhaler, try this: put food into your mouth, chew it really well, and then swallow it before you put the next mouthful in. I know that sounds simple, but try it. It can take an enormous amount of concentration for food inhalers to change their eating behaviours. It might help to put your fork or spoon down between each mouthful, or engage in conversation if you are eating with others. Or think of your own technique to slow yourself down if you shovel your food in. You need to pay attention when you eat to how you eat and in my ideal world you would only eat in a calm environment. I appreciate this is not always possible but if this is an area you want to work on, do all you can to eat in calm surroundings.

KEEP AN EYE ON PORTION SIZE

Now, back to the stomach, the first place food lands after you have swallowed it. Clench your fist and look at it. That is how big your stomach is without any food in it. Tiny, isn't it? Now think about what happens when you pile your plate high in the evening and inhale that big mountain of food. Your stomach has to stretch to accommodate it. And then the food has to sit in the stomach for a minimum of thirty minutes to allow the stomach acid and other digestive juices to really begin to break the food down.

It makes sense that eating too much total food can lead to a bloated stomach and digestive system problems. A rough guide to the amount of food we need to eat at each meal is approximately two fist sizes of concentrated food such as proteins or carbohydrates. You can, and need to, add as many greens (non-starch vegetables and/or salad) to that as you like. Although they have a very high nutrient content, they are mostly water.

Many people know that they need to reduce their portion size or not eat more food after dinner, yet no matter how hard they seem to try, they can't seem to eat less or stop eating once they start. It always comes back to the why.

STOMACH ACID IS A GOOD THING

Food arrives at the stomach after you have chewed and swallowed it. But even before you take a bite, the aroma of food can stimulate the production of stomach acid, an exceptionally important substance when it comes to great digestion. The role of the stomach acid is to break food down. Imagine your food is a big long string of circles as shown in the first row of the diagram below. It is the job of the stomach acid to go chop, chop, chop and break the circles apart into smaller bunches, as the second row illustrates.

0000000000000000000000
⇓ (stomach acid)
000 00 000 000 00 0000 00

Digestion: *The action of stomach acid on whole foods breaks them down into their smaller components.*

Your body is governed by pH ranges. In scientific terms pH refers to the concentration of hydrogen ions present; it is a measure of acidity or alkalinity. The pH range is based on a scale from 1 to 14, with 1 being the acid end of the spectrum and 14 being the alkaline end, while 7 is neutral. Every fluid, every tissue, every cell of your body has a pH level at which it performs optimally. For example, the optimal pH of stomach acid is 1.9, which is so acidic it would burn you if it touched your skin. But it won't while it is nicely housed inside your stomach, as the cells that line the stomach itself not only produce stomach acid but are also designed to withstand the super acidic conditions.

For many women though, the pH level of the stomach acid is not acidic *enough*, and it may have a pH far greater than 1.9, which is not ideal for digestion. To be precise, animal proteins are optimally digested at a pH of 1.9, while starch is optimally digested at a pH of 2.1. This may not seem like much of a difference, but inside your body it can mean the difference between a flat abdomen and one that is bloated after a meal.

REFLUX AND INDIGESTION

Adults with reflux or indigestion tend to assume that the burning sensation they experience with heartburn means they are producing too much acid when the reality is usually the opposite. They are usually not making enough stomach acid and/or the pH of it is too high. To understand this, remember the food as a string of circles analogy and that stomach acid plays a vital role in breaking the circles apart. A pH that is much higher than 1.9 cannot effectively break the circles apart, leaving larger, undigested segments that cannot be further broken down to continue along the digestive tract. Rather than allowing that food to proceed down into the small intestine for the next part of its journey, the body regurgitates the food in an attempt to get rid of it. You then experience the acid burn and assume it is *too* acidic when in fact it is not acidic enough to break the food down properly and allow it to pass into the small intestine. It "burns" you because anything with an acid pH that is too acidic for the tissue to which it is exposed will create a burning sensation. When the acid is contained inside the stomach pouch, all is well, but when it escapes out of this area, it affects the lining of the esophagus and the first part of the small intestine, which are not designed to cope with such acidic contents. Many people with reflux respond very well to the stimulation of stomach acid and/or to omitting foods that are a problem for them and experience much fewer symptoms as a result. I have met countless people whose reflux symptoms completely resolved after omitting either dairy products (precisely omitting the casein) and/or gluten, a protein found in the grains wheat, rye, barley, triticale, and oats, although oats have a low level. Incredibly, a number of these people had experienced such severe reflux in the past that they had surgery in an attempt to resolve it. When this didn't work, they believed nothing would ever relieve it, not even medication. They were beyond thrilled when dietary change solved it. Your body has a wisdom far beyond your mind. It knows better than your taste buds what it wants and what is good for you. And it will let you know this if you choose to pay attention.

I do meet people who describe specific foods affecting their reflux but not every time they consume them, and granted this can be a little more of a challenge to solve. However, with this health scenario, it seems to be the combination of the aggravating food with the hormonal and nervous system scenarios communicating to the body that they need to be on red alert rather than digesting food. I'll get to this in a moment as this same combination can present as the symptoms for IBS or simply a bloated abdomen.

HOW TO GET YOUR STOMACH ACID GOING

Stomach acid production is stimulated by the aroma

of food and by chewing, but also by the consumption of lemon juice and apple cider vinegar. Historically, we used to take much longer to prepare our meals and the aromas of the upcoming meal generated by slower cooking processes signalled to the stomach that food was on its way. Chewing also alerts the brain to send a message to the stomach to let it know that food is on its way. When we inhale our food, however, this doesn't happen. Another way to physically stimulate the production of stomach acid is by taking lemon juice and apple cider vinegar. If you haven't consumed either of these before, it is initially best to dilute them and, ideally, consume them five to twenty minutes before breakfast (or all of your main meals if that appeals). For example, you might begin with half a teaspoon of apple cider vinegar in as much water as you like. Over the coming days and weeks, gradually work up to having one tablespoon of apple cider vinegar while at the same time you gradually decrease the amount of water. If you prefer lemon juice, start with the juice of half a lemon diluted with warm water to your taste, and then gradually work up to having the juice of a whole lemon in less warm water. (As an aside, it is a good idea to brush your teeth after your meals when you use lemon in order to prevent any potential problems with tooth enamel.) Use these tips to wake your stomach acid up before you eat.

IT'S BEST NOT TO DRINK WATER WITH MEALS

For the most effective digestion and to help prevent bloating, we need the pH of our stomach acid to sit at around 2. Water has a pH of 7 (neutral pH) or above, depending on the mineral content (the higher the mineral content, the higher/more alkaline the pH level). When you add a liquid with a pH of 7 or more to one with a pH of 2, what do you potentially do to the stomach acid? You dilute it. And we need all of the digestive fire we can muster to get the maximum nourishment from our food and the best out of us. So, in my ideal world, we wouldn't drink water thirty minutes either side of eating. Aim to drink *water* between meals, not with meals. It can be a challenging habit to break. Set yourself a goal of not drinking with meals for one week… and then try to keep the new habit going. Or add a squeeze of fresh lemon juice if you insist on water with your meal. Just cut it out for a week, one little week out of your very long life, and see if you feel any different.

HOW PH LEVELS RUN YOUR DIGESTIVE SYSTEM

Once food has been somewhat broken down in the stomach, it moves through the pyloric sphincter, a one-way valve leading into the duodenum, the beginning of the small intestine. In your body this valve is located in the middle (or just slightly on the left) of the chest, just below your bra.

While food is in the stomach, messages are being sent to the pancreas to secrete sodium bicarbonate (as well as digestive enzymes), which has a highly alkaline pH. The bicarbonate is designed to protect the lining of the first part of the small intestine as well as to allow digestion to continue. What is known as a "pH gradient" is established all the way along the digestive tract, and each region of the big, long tube has an ideal pH. When the pH gradient is not established in the stomach, that is, when the pH is higher than ideal, digestion problems are likely further along the tract. These may be symptoms of the small or large intestine, such as bloating, pain, or excessive gas. A less than ideal pH gradient means that the absorption of nutrients may be compromised as well. Insufficient pancreatic bicarbonate production may also cause digestive symptoms such as a burning sensation underneath the stomach in the valve area described above. Pain in this area can also indicate that the gall bladder needs some support or investigation. It is best to consult with your health-care professional about this if you feel discomfort in this area.

The best way to let the pancreas know that it needs to jump into action and produce bicarbonate and digestive enzymes is to have good stomach acid production at optimal pH. The digestive system runs off a cascade of signals from one organ or area to the next, via the brain. Use the strategies I've suggested, especially chewing food well, to stimulate the pancreas to fulfil its role.

There have been occasions when I have suggested clients use supplements of pancreatic enzymes; this is appropriate if there is a genuine lack of these enzymes rather than simply poor stomach acid conditions. I usually suggest the strategies before trialling supplements; however, when symptoms are severe and once other causes have been ruled out, a gastroenterologist may measure pancreatic enzyme levels.

ABSORBING THE GOODNESS

The small intestine is where absorption of most of the nutrients in the food you eat begins. As food moves through the small bowel, digestive enzymes are secreted not only by the pancreas but also from the lining of the small intestine. The role of these enzymes is to continue what the stomach acid began, which is to continue to break down the food we have eaten into its smallest, most basic components. It is in the small intestine that you absorb most of the goodness (vitamins and minerals) from your food.

Think about that. All of the goodness, all of the nutrients that keep you alive are drawn out of your food and into your blood so that your body can use those nutrients to do all of the life-sustaining jobs they do. Alcohol and vitamin B12 are virtually the only substances you absorb directly out of your stomach (rather than your small intestine) into your blood. Alcohol tends to be in your blood within five minutes of consuming it, which is why people may get tipsy if they drink it on an empty stomach.

The small intestine is where the nutrients in your food move from the tube that is your digestive tract into the blood, which is obviously a different set of tubes. This is how we are nourished, and it is how you stay alive.

Just because you eat something, though, doesn't mean you get all of the goodness out of it. If a food contains, for example, ten milligrams of zinc, you're unlikely to absorb the whole ten milligrams when you eat it. The absorption of nutrients is dependent on a whole host of factors, some still to be discussed, while some of which have been discussed above: if you inhale your food, drink water with your meals, or have poor stomach acid production, for example, you may absorb very little of the goodness in your food. Think that through: nutrients are essential for life and simply as a result of *the way* you are eating, let alone the foods you might be choosing, you might be robbing yourself of some of the goodness your food provides. Give yourself the best opportunity to absorb as much goodness out of your food as possible by applying the tips above! It may add energy to your years and years to your life.

GUT BACTERIA CAN BE YOUR FRIENDS—AND YOUR ENEMIES

Now that the food has progressed through to the large intestine, can you guess what lives in here? Bacteria. On average, an adult will have two to four kilograms (four to nine pounds) of bacteria living in their colon. So, just as an aside, every time you weigh yourself remember that two to four of the kilos you see in that number on the scales is made up of gut bacteria that are essential for life. See how crazy it is that you weigh yourself? All you do when you weigh yourself is weigh your self-esteem.

Some of the bacteria in your large bowel (colon) are good guys and some are bad guys. Obviously, you want more good guys than bad guys. The role of the gut bacteria is to ferment whatever you give them. To come back to the circle concept of food illustrated previously, gut bugs love it when you give them something that is one or even two circles in size. They know what to do with that. But if a previous digestive process has not been completed sufficiently, the gut bacteria in your colon may be presented with fragments of food that are five or even seven circles in size, and all they know to do with any food they are offered is to ferment it.

What word springs to mind when you think of fermentation? I love asking this question at my seminars, as the answers usually amuse me as well as the other audience members. People will often say "beer," "wine," "sauerkraut"! But usually in the end I get the answer I'm after, which is gas. Fermentation involves bacterial action on a food source and the subsequent production of gas. Some gases are essential to the health of the cells that line our gut, while others seem to irritate the gut and cause a bloated, uncomfortable stomach as the day progresses, whether we have eaten in a "healthy" way or not.

The trouble with a bloated stomach for so many women is that it messes with their brain. When they look down and see a swollen tummy, something inside immediately communicates to every cell of their body that they are fat, whether it's something they consciously think or not. Many of my clients go up a size around the waist as the day progresses even though they feel they have eaten with their health in mind. This occurrence can add a layer of stress to a woman's life that they just don't need. It is especially stressful because they can't fathom why it is happening. Sometimes it is the foods you choose. Sometimes it is the bugs that live in your colon. Sometimes it is because of poor digestion further up the process such as insufficient stomach acid production. In traditional Chinese medicine (TCM), this is considered a spleen and/or liver picture and a TCM practitioner is likely to use acupuncture and/or herbs to support these organs. In metaphysical medicine, there is something in your world that you cannot "digest" and there is a fear that you are yet to resolve.

HOW STRESS PLAYS HAVOC WITH YOUR DIGESTION

When it comes to poor digestion, IBS, or simply a bloated tummy, other than food or a parasite infection (discussed in a moment), stress is a major contributing factor.

The body has your best interests at heart. When you make adrenalin, and your sympathetic nervous system is firing that you need to be sustaining the fight or flight response, the last thing your body wants is for you to perhaps recall that it has been a few hours since you last ate and be distracted by food when you need to remain focused on getting away from whatever is "threatening" you rather than on securing your next meal. And to power your escape your blood supply is diverted away from your digestive system to your periphery, to your arms and your legs. And so when the food arrives when you are in this state, your body does not have the resources to digest it. It is in fight or flight (SNS dominance) when it needs to be in rest and digest (PNS dominance) to do this vital work.

So if you have had sinister bowel diseases ruled out, yet you have what has been diagnosed as IBS or a bloated tummy, and you have tried every dietary change under the sun properly to no avail (and I say "properly" as I meet countless women who tell me they cut out gluten, for example, to see if this would make a difference to their digestion problems and when they tell me that it didn't make a difference but that they didn't stop eating sandwiches for lunch because they are convenient… well they haven't yet done a proper gluten free diet!) and you have used herbs to resolve any potential gut bacteria/parasite problem and you still have your symptoms, then I encourage you to see your digestive system symptoms as a wake-up call. It is your body crying out for you to treat yourself differently. It is time to stop trying, to stop coming up with strategies that will "fix" you. It is time to be. And you will need to schedule time to simply be if you have a full life. It is time to honour the gut feelings you have and trust your intuition. This is a journey from your head to your heart. It is time to stop running (literally and figuratively) and remember that you are not your past, you are not your stories, and that it, whatever it is, can no longer hurt you unless you allow that. It is time to fully appreciate that you are wonderful and that you are loved, just the way you are.

WHAT IS A LEAKY GUT?

An additional concept within digestive health that is not only fascinating but has wide-ranging effects on how we feel and function—including gut transit time (how quickly food moves through the digestive system), mood, concentration, behaviour and, potentially, food addictions—is a concept known as leaky gut.

The cells that line a healthy small intestine look like a row of neatly stacked bricks with finger-like projections (called "villi"), side by side as demonstrated in the picture below.

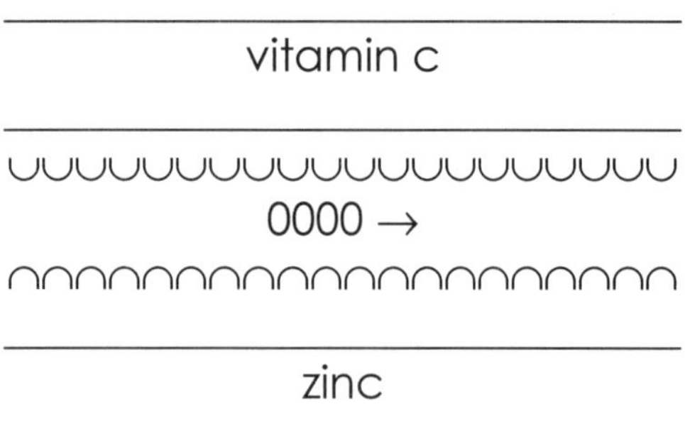

A Healthy Gut: *Food (circles) travelling through a healthy mature intestine moves straight ahead. Only nutrients (e.g. Vitamin C and zinc) enter the blood vessels that closely follow the intestines.*

In a healthy gut, only the tiny *nutrients* (vitamins and minerals) diffuse (move) through the gut wall into the blood, and this is the precious process through which we are nourished and stay alive. However, the cells that line the gut can come apart, as if the bricks are stacked with gaps, illustrated below. This is, in fact, how we are born.

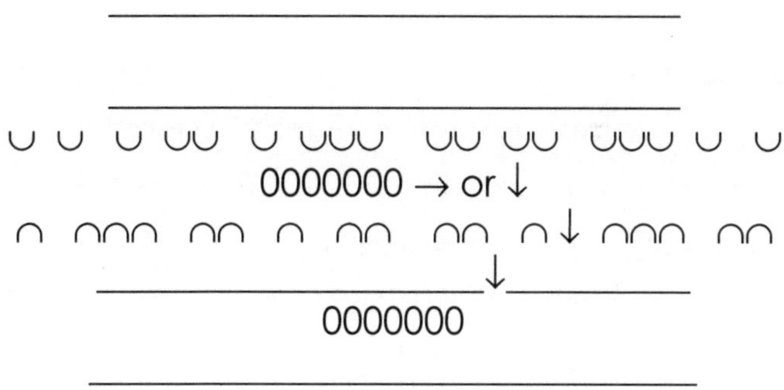

A "Leaky" Gut: *Food (circles) travels through an immature gut or a "leaky" intestine. Microscopic, poorly digested fragments of food can escape out of the gut and enter the blood.*

When we are born, the cells that line our digestive system are a distance apart, which is why we can't feed all foods to newborns; foods must be gradually introduced to a child over time to prevent allergic reactions as the gut matures. The gut is immature when we are born, and it slowly matures from birth until reaching full maturity somewhere between the ages of two and five, depending on the individual child and their health and life experiences in the early years. The cells that line the gut can, however, also come apart during adulthood as a result of the exaggerated production of a protein called zonulin (explored in a moment), gastrointestinal infection, or stress. The chronic production of stress hormones can compromise the integrity of the gut cells and signal to them that they need to move further apart so that more nutrition can get through to the blood, as nutrient requirements increase during times of stress. Everything about us is geared for survival. Trouble is, and as you now understand, we can get stuck in this stress response.

When food travels through a gut with good cell lining integrity, it can only go straight ahead. However, if it travels through a gut in which the cells have come apart, it may go straight ahead, or it may move out of the gut and into the blood. Fragments of food are not intended to enter the blood. Nutrients, the vitamins and minerals from food, are; but if actual fragments of food enter the bloodstream, the immune system, which is what protects you from infection, thinks that the food fragment is a germ and it mounts an immune response against it. This is one way adults develop food sensitivities. Poor gut integrity is also described as "leaky gut."

Once you were able to eat anything without a

problem, and now certain foods seem to cause you grief. This process can be healed by minimizing the irritation to the gut lining, which can mean avoiding some foods or ingredients for a period of time while also working on the gut integrity. Once we've worked out why someone has "leaky gut" symptoms in the first place, they will often be able to tolerate the foods that caused them irritation. Did the problem begin as a result of stress or an infection? The power to heal the symptoms is always in the why, so think about your road in.

The blood supply into which the food fragments flow is the same blood supply that goes to your brain. Humans have what is known as the blood-brain barrier (BBB), a semi-permeable layer separating the peripheral blood supply from that of the brain. The BBB was always considered to be a highly selective membrane that only allowed substances into the brain that would be of benefit. Research has now shown us that this is not the case. In cases where gut permeability is increased, the BBB is often suspected of having the same increased permeability.

LEAKY GUTS, BLOATED TUMMIES, AND FOOD ADDICTION

If we could literally see the food fragments, we'd see their structure is very similar to that of opioids.

Opioids are substances that help humans feel good. They also modulate pain. Our natural feel-good hormones have an opioid-based structure and are called endorphins. In our brains and in our guts, we have what are called opioid receptors. Just because your body makes a substance (a hormone, for example) doesn't mean you necessarily get the effects of that substance. It must bind to a receptor for you to get the effect generated by that hormone. In this case, when we make endorphins and they bind to the opioid receptors, we feel pleasure. Heroin and morphine are also opioids and they too bind to the opioid receptors in the brain. Anything that gives a human pleasure has the potential to be addictive, which is why humans can be addicted to these drugs. You can also see how someone might become addicted to exercise since activity certainly generates endorphins. So, whatever spins your tyres—a sunset, a spin class, a particular fragrance or song, or a child's laughter—what happens in that moment is that you have made endorphins, they have bound to opioid receptors, and you have felt pleasure.

But how does this relate to digestion, food, rushing, and stress? Some of the fragments of food that can escape out of a leaky gut into the bloodstream can also have an opioid structure. Their names include beta-casomorphine and gluteo-morphine and they are partially digested fragments of casein, the major protein in cow's milk products, and gluten from the grains mentioned earlier. Just like endorphins, these opioids from food have the capacity to bind to the opioid receptors in the brain and very subtly make us feel good. The effect is not usually noticed as an enormous boost in mood, but the person will often feel they can't live without the food, and they find they'll *have to* eat it in some form daily or even at every meal.

I have seen this to be the case with countless clients. While some people have no problem omitting a food from their diet for a trial period when they have a set of symptoms that warrants it, others will beg me not to take them off the food. This is despite the fact they are seeing me because they want to sort out their problematic bowels, and all I am asking is that they omit a particular food for four measly weeks, something that may just give them the answer to some of their health concerns! I am not judging someone who responds in this way. I am simply pointing out to you that the power food can have over an individual is just like an addiction. Their connection to it, their need for it, is often highly emotional and also potentially physical through this opioid mechanism.

TRADITIONAL CHINESE MEDICINE AND THE SPLEEN

According to traditional Chinese medicine, the spleen rules digestion. Traditional Chinese medicine considers that each organ has its own vital energy as well as there being whole-body energy. If spleen energy is down, you will feel your usual hunger for meals, but as soon as you eat even a small amount, you will feel full and possibly bloated. Your short-term memory is likely to not be what it once was, and you may possibly feel like you eat like a bird yet your clothes continue to get tighter. According to traditional Chinese medicine, when you present with this health picture they may suggest that your spleen energy is low.

Stimulating spleen energy can make a real difference. Acupuncture will do this, as will bitter herbs. Spleen energy can result from what is simply described as overthinking. According to Chinese medicine, the busy mind, relentlessly thinking of the next thing you need to do, takes energy away from the vital process of digestion every day. The spleen may also lose some of its strength if your liver or kidney (the adrenal glands, makers of adrenalin, sit on top of the kidneys) energy is overbearing or low. Working with a wonderful practitioner of TCM can assist you in healing your gut, and many additional digestive system remedies are offered in the solutions chapter.

ZONULIN AND GUT INTEGRITY

In 2000, a new protein made inside the body was discovered (by a researcher called Dr Fasano if you want to read about it further). Named zonulin, it is a physiological modulator of what are called the intracellular tight junctions of the gut. Put simply, zonulin plays a role in whether the cells that line the gut are neatly packed together or if they come apart and "leak." Researchers originally thought, for example, that coeliac (celiac) disease, a condition in which gluten drives the immune system to attack the villi that line the small intestine, only involved gluten and genes. What they have since discovered is that zonulin is at a minimum thirty times higher in people with coeliac disease, even when they have been on a gluten-free diet for two years, than those without coeliac disease, even if they have gut symptoms. What in broad terms can be called "bad" gut bugs such as *Salmonella* have been shown to stimulate zonulin production (which would increase gut permeability/leakiness) and that the presence of these bad bugs enhances gluten's capacity to cause damage to the lining of the intestine; while good bacteria such as *Bifidus* bacteria have been shown to virtually eliminate gluten's ability to cause damage. As an aside, research is currently being done exploring the role of zonulin, increased gut permeability, and the development of autoimmune diseases such as multiple sclerosis and lupus. We have to wait and see what the outcomes will be, but I can say for certain that the gut is incredibly crucial to our health.

I include this information here for a few reasons. Firstly, I wanted to highlight that science is constantly teaching us more and more about the gut and that is a wonderful thing. I believe that in the big scheme of things we know very little about the enormous multitude of roles gut bacteria play in our health. And I wanted to suggest that it is likely that problems with gut bacteria are contributing to the significant increase in gut-based health problems we are seeing. This is partly, I believe, due to the effect of rushing, as I've outlined above, with the cascade of hormone and nervous system events leading to poor digestion. And sadly, I believe it may also be the result of the ongoing presence of antibiotics in the food supply. In the United States alone the Federal Drug Administration (FDA) estimates that the amount of antimicrobial drugs sold and distributed for use in food animals is 13.1 million kilograms (28.8 million pounds) per year (2008 data) while approximately

3.3 million kilos (just over 7 million pounds) were sold for human use (2009 data). Sure the rest of the world's consumption is smaller and there are many countries around the world who rigidly (wonderfully) regulate the use of antibiotics in animals, but I simply wanted to point out that if the animals get the antibiotic, there will be residue in their tissues if humans eat it. I believe in the long term, this is then having an effect on the gut bacteria profiles of humans and changing our digestive systems. One of the reasons I believe this is that over the past fourteen years, I have observed (OK, so this is not based on scientific research, but it is my observation as a health professional) that almost the only people who don't have gut problems are long-term vegans.

I am not suggesting you all become vegans, unless this resonates for you. I am simply offering you an explanation about why so many women have gut problems today. The combination of stress and the changing gut bacteria profiles is playing a significant role. Please become aware of how much meat you eat, where it comes from, what the animals were fed, and how they were raised, if not for their sake then for yours. Please choose organically-reared, pasture-fed meat. The farmers supply what consumers demand. So you can slowly change the world through how you spend your money. There is now significant scientific evidence that a diet high in plant-based foods not only prevents a significant amount of degenerative disease but can also reverse some of the damage once illnesses such as type 2 diabetes, high blood pressure and heart disease have been diagnosed. Imagine your diet being so powerful.

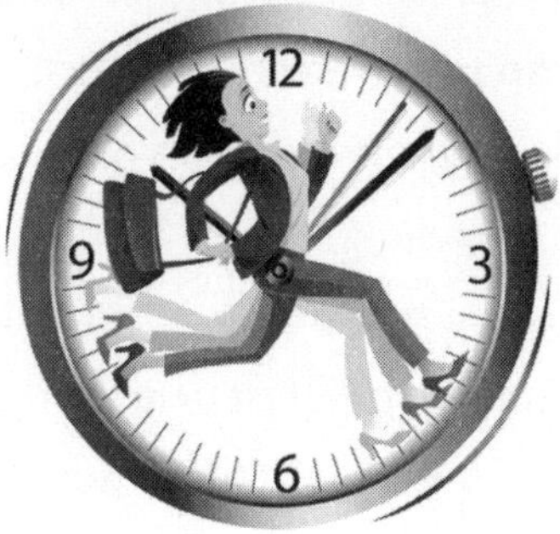

Chapter 5

The Emotional Perspective:

lifting the veil between behaviour and beliefs

This section of Rushing Woman's Syndrome offers you the opportunity to literally get to the heart of your matter—to the heart of why you feel the need to run your life with urgency, why you have chosen, and I don't say that lightly, to do what you do and fill your days and nights the way you do. In all honesty, this is my favourite part of what I do because this is where behavioural change is sustained rather than temporary. This is the part that allows you to rest the part of you that is weary and awaken the part of you that is asleep. And optimal health on every level—physical, emotional, and spiritual—is then on offer to you.

BELIEFS AND BEHAVIOURS

Every human's greatest fear is that they are not enough and as a result that they won't be loved. We are born this way. It is human psychology 101. Without love a human baby dies. Other animals won't. So this is not some artificial construct that develops over time—it is hardwired into us at our most fundamental level.

Yet as adults, a life jam-packed with love is delicious but not essential to our survival. When we live as if love is crucial to our survival, and we do anything and everything we can to avoid ever being rejected, we live our lives as if we are still a child. The trouble is most of us have no idea that this is what we are doing. We don't realise that the reason we went back to the fridge after a filling dinner last night was to avoid feeling rejected. We've blanketed that with a story that we simply feel like it, or we deserve it having worked so hard all day. But human behaviour is the outermost expression of our inner beliefs. It is that simple. Think about that: human behaviour is the outermost expression of our inner beliefs and yet most of us absorbed a set of beliefs before we were old enough to think for ourselves. And, unless we question these beliefs, they become the default lenses through which we view every situation we ever encounter.

Before our current era of urgency due to the immediacy of the ways many people expect themselves and others to function and communicate—via mobile phones that they are never without, emails that people expect a reply to within minutes, supermarkets that gather food items together, having every last thing you want in stock, immediate answers to questions via a Google search, social media posts requiring responses 24/7—our outermost expressions of not being enough, not being loved, and being rejected, played out in the way we ate, the way we spent money, and the way we spoke to the people around us (to name but a few). In fact, they still do. Yet, in this age of Google speed, there is now another more obvious, more intense and, in my opinion, potentially even more damaging way that this belief is playing out—and that is with women living out the perception that they have to be all things to all people so that they will never, ever be rejected, even though they have no idea that is what they are doing. And to fit everything in, to do all they "have" to do so that they never, ever let anyone down and risk being "rejected," they have gone into overdrive. Otherwise, why would you do it, unless somewhere inside you, you perceived that your life depended on it? Seriously. As I love to say, it's always about love. Everything always is.

My favourite author Geneen Roth says, "We all follow life instructions given to us ten or thirty or fifty years ago by people we wouldn't ask street directions from today." We created meanings from what was going on around us at a very young age, only we don't know this is what we were doing. We simply thought that when Dad had "that" look on his face, it meant he was happy or sad or angry or about to explode. And when Mum made "that" sigh sound, it meant that she was disappointed or tired or relieved. We created those meanings. In these situations, our mother and father hadn't told us with words that they felt a certain way. We observed them and the environment and formed beliefs about how the world is. Yet this is *our* version of the world, which is why, when you speak to twins about their lives growing up, you can wonder whether they have come from the same family.

I've listed some examples below to help you make sense of this concept. "Don't be so full of yourself; people don't like that" can eventually, if we hear it enough times, become the belief that "if I want to be loved and accepted, I need to dull and dim and dumb myself down." Another example... If we see our parents arguing about money, if money is a source of conflict in our families, or if no one ever talks about it, we give meaning to those situations in the form of beliefs: "If I want to be happy in a relationship, I'd better not talk about, not think about, not ever bring up the subject of money."

We understand situations by giving them meaning. And out of these meanings beliefs are created, which once formed, become the template for how we see ourselves and how we behave. We then spend the rest of our lives acting as if our subjective beliefs—I will never have enough, I must keep the peace, I am lazy/dumb/unlovable, if I'm not slim/wealthy/a yes-girl I won't be loved—are reality itself. We believe that the way we see our situation is the way things are and that there is no other way. And our actions follow accordingly. Most of us don't even know what we believe. We are convinced of the rightness of what we see and feel, that we don't realize that we see things as *we* are, not as they are. It never occurs to us that our belief system is subjective, that there are dozens of ways to interpret the same situation and as Geneen so beautifully says "unless we name and recognize the extent to which our own version of reality is based on instructions given to us by people we wouldn't ask for street directions today, our emotional, financial and spiritual lives will remain frozen in the past, hijacked by beliefs that, for the most part, are out of alignment with, and have no relevance to, our current ideals and values and the adults we've become."

As much as I love positivity and optimism—I consider myself to have both of those traits—I have not found that it is possible to completely replace one set of beliefs with another by only using what have become known as "affirmations." Of course they can help. They help shift your focus to one of positivity and help you have hope that life can be better. But you can repeat "I am lovable" a thousand times a day, you can put "I am super successful" in your car, on your mirror, your computer screen, inside your glasses if you like, but if an earlier belief or conviction of being unlovable is installed in your psyche based on beliefs you created before you could talk, you will only feel better for a moment because you won't actually believe yourself. If you don't do the actual work of deconstructing your fundamental beliefs, the affirmations have no place to land or stick, and their impact is unlikely to be lasting. Please don't get me wrong. By all means do affirmations. They can be nourishment for your soul. I'm simply saying that I have yet to meet someone for whom they alone dismantled what was laid down at the beginning of their time on earth. Of course be positive and affirm that you are loved. Just explore your beliefs as well for lasting, sustained change.

When people say things like "Your beliefs determine your experience," think about this... if you believe that there aren't enough hours in the day or if you believe in being poor or that you will always be fat, that will be your experience. In other words when you look through "shattered" lenses, the world looks "shattered." It has always been true that you act according to your beliefs and, since the way you act has consequences, your beliefs manifest in the world through various situations. When you act out your beliefs, you see the results of your actions everywhere. It is precisely what happens when you buy a certain coloured car of a specific make and model... you suddenly see those cars everywhere! Well guess what? They've always been there. It is simply that now your eyes are primed to notice them. Beliefs work the same way. You see "evidence" of what you believe everywhere, and you never notice the zillions of examples that make those beliefs null and void.

Clearly it is taking different actions, not just naming beliefs, that leads to change, but in my experience with human health, achieving long-lasting change is impossible without first becoming aware of the deep-seated convictions that are driving your behaviour. If you don't realize that the way you are seeing things is not the way they are, if you don't understand that you see yourself, your family, your relationships with food, money, and the world through a version of reality that you developed before you could talk, you believe there is no other way to see and consider the world. You only know what you have experienced and therefore those around you must be hallucinating if they describe it any other way.

EXPECTATIONS AND URGENCY

I've witnessed the change in people's expectations over the past five years in my practice. Many expect one ninety minute nutrition-focussed consultation to "fix" their entire lives, when they've been using food to cope for at least 15,768,000 minutes (thirty years). You gotta peel back the layers of the onion through kindness and curiosity about what led you to this point, yet most of you believe the only way to sort out your body, for example, is to deprive yourself and work harder and that if you can't do this then you are a failure before you've even begun.

I've witnessed the massive efforts women make in thousands of clients. They cannot eat any better, even by my exceptionally high nutritional standards.

They cannot move any more than they are already, and their clothes keep getting tighter and tighter. They cannot (until I guide them there) "see" that there are other ways for bodies to grow or shrink than the calorie equation they have been bombarded with for their entire lives: eat less, move more. My book *Accidentally Overweight* explores precisely this concept: that there is more to fat loss than just calories. If your body gets the message for sixteen hours a day, day after day, that your life is in danger and that you must be prepared to run or fight at any moment, your body won't want to use your fat as fuel. Calming down is the first step for so many women. They need to change the way they eat, exercise, live, think, and behave to ways based on calm. Yet when I explain to them that this panic, this haste, this urgency is what has to change first, many stare at me blankly like I've just asked them to repeat third form algebra or recite Latin phrases backwards that they've long forgotten. "What do you mean slowing down will change everything? That means I'll get less done in a day, and you clearly don't understand the pressure I'm under. I run a small country called my life!" "What do you mean do yoga instead of marathon training—you've got to be crazy—I can't lose weight burning all of the calories I burn doing all of this running… I'll become the size of a house if I 'only do yoga.'" And yet doing the same thing day after day and expecting a different outcome has become known as a definition of insanity. It is time to do it differently and take care of your health in the process.

HOW TO "DO" THE SLOW DOWN

Many women have no idea how to slow down. And when I tell them they actually just have to be, after all we are human beings rather than human doings, I can see from the look on their face that they do their best to hide, that they'd rather go and put their head in a bucket of ice water—that would be easier than surrendering.

So I give them things to do. I offer women ways to bring calm and spaciousness back into their lives. And get them thoroughly exploring, with kindness and curiosity, rather than judgment, what has lead them to relentlessly pursue whatever it is that they think they want. You have to do that bit. But then you have to go further. Because it is not about having whatever it is… a larger bank balance, no mortgage, thinner thighs… it is about your perception of how having these things will make you feel. And I am yet to have one single client not pull her veil back and see that, after all, it really is love she is chasing (even though she may or may not already have a life full of love). And in that moment, I always have tears rolling down my face because I know her life will never be the same again. Because in that moment, she has caught a glimpse that what she has been searching for, relentlessly pursuing, is actually within her. And stillness and calm allow you to see it and feel it. She was born that way. She simply forgot. And she will likely forget again, only next time, for not as long. And the strategies help with that. And they make up the final chapter.

So yes, as I said, one definition of insanity is doing the same thing over and over, year after year, and expecting a different outcome. Yet it is like we are in a trance for ten or thirty years or, for a some, a lifetime, *doing* all we can to make ourselves "more," as if we are not enough, yet not seeing that we just keep doing the same thing over and over and our lives never seem to look any different. We think we just require a different diet, or a different exercise program, or less food on our plate, and that will make all the difference. What women need first is to stop dieting.

Here is a piece I wrote for a magazine about why diets don't work and I include it here so you can understand the science and also the psychology behind a topic that can be a huge source of stress for women.

Why Diets Don't Work

It is well-known that the majority of

people who go on diets end up regaining any weight they lose plus more—83 percent in fact—and they regain it within a two-year period. At the heart of this effect is a precise scientific process which on the surface may appear harmless, yet underneath, it is a yo-yo cycle that bounces between strict deprivation and a free-for-all with food. If people try to lose weight by shaming and depriving themselves, weight loss will not necessarily occur; they simply end up shamed and deprived.

Biochemically there is a stress hormone called cortisol that the adrenal glands make. Historically the only time humans made cortisol were scenarios of physical stress where food was scarce such as floods, famines, and wars. People with the highest levels of body fat tended to survive these times so cortisol acted to slow down metabolic rate and communicate to the body that it needed to store fat. Even though we live in a modern world our subconscious biochemical reactions to chronic stress are the same as they were historically, even though we may think differently and our subconscious mind, running our lives 95 percent of the time, is one million times more powerful than our conscious mind.

Over the past two decades, the human body has been asked to change at a rate greater than at any other time in history;

a rate I have come to call "Google speed." With the advent of the Internet, cell phones, email, and social media, we are amped up and on call 24/7. Today, chronic stress, hence cortisol production, tends to come from long-term psychological worries about relationships, finances, health issues, or body shape, size, and weight. We have forgotten how essential it is to every aspect of our health, including our body size, to just switch off, rest, and activate vital restorative processes.

We also tend to make cortisol when we "starve" ourselves. If you suddenly go from overeating food to not eating very much food at all, your body tends to make cortisol because it doesn't understand that you have just embarked on a diet. It thinks there is no food left in the world so it has no choice but to try to save your life and to do this, it slows your metabolism right down. So then when you stop dieting and you return to the way you used to eat, which you will unless you have truly explored what is at the heart of your matter, you will not just return to the size you once were, you will naturally grow beyond that as your metabolism will have slowed down.

Many people attempt to address this by exercising fanatically yet when you do this, your body can perceive it is fleeing from danger and subconsciously activate the message that it is caught up in the "floods, famines, and war" scenario, receiving the biochemical message that to be "safe" it still needs to store fat rather than burn it.

What do most people do when their clothes get tight? They go on a what? A diet. And when you go on a diet, do you eat more or less? Usually less yet and when you do this, you simply confirm to your body what it perceives to be true (what cortisol is communicating); that there is limited food left in the world when, in fact, food is likely to be abundant for you.

With any system that addresses weight, unless it also explores what is literally at the heart of someone's matter rather than the size of their thighs, it won't work, and any diet that may lead to weight loss initially but where the weight is regained, is not a successful diet. I meet people every day who say the X diet worked for them. Yet there they are in front of me physically bigger than they were before they went on the X diet so, no, actually the X diet did not work for them. If someone has gone on a diet, lost weight, and kept it off, a far deeper shift has happened within them to foster that sustained change. Because guess what... and what I'm about to say may surprise you coming from a nutrition expert... it is not about the food.

At the heart of any addiction, whether that is an addiction to food itself or simply an addiction to constantly judging yourself based on the size and shape of your body, regardless of its shape and size, is the belief in your own deficiency and the assumption that it can be fixed with an external substance or regime.

People eat unresourcefully for many reasons. It can be a biochemical reason such as low blood glucose that leads someone to polish off too many sweet foods for afternoon tea, or it can be emotional, such as when someone creates a meaning of rejection when a colleague gives them constructive feedback at work and they soothe their hurt with food. Or it can be both. Mostly it is both.

So now you can truly appreciate why diets don't work, due to both biochemical and emotional factors. Despite the latest fad being purported as the ultimate weight-loss solution, they simply offer short-term results for a long-term additional gain. Lasting weight loss is never achieved with a fad that starves your body and your soul.

~~~~~~~~~~~~~~~

SELF-REFLECTION

A client recently shared this with me:

> *"One major thing I've learnt since working with you is that I've never really done any self-reflection or looked at why I do the things I do. I thought I was too busy, well at*
~~~~~~~~~~~~~~~

least that's the way I perceived it. I thought my answers would be in some pill, website, magazine, or person. It is so easy to direct the focus away from asking yourself hard-hitting questions, but actually only in the short term. When I've looked at myself in the mirror sometimes, I've thought it's as if the lights are on but no one's home. I once had to go to a meeting and they'd phoned the day before to confirm I was coming and to let me know I couldn't park in the car park, yet I still parked in the car park only a day later. It's as if I was hearing words but I'd lost the ability to really listen and process the information. I was getting appointment dates and times wrong because I'd come to rely on someone texting me to remind me that I have a hair appointment so if they didn't text me, I didn't turn up. It was as if I couldn't remember any details because my mind was fried by all I felt I had to achieve in a day."

This gorgeous lady took a journey from her head to her heart. It was the shortest distance she ever travelled yet she resisted for some time, denying, unable to see her outward expressions of a cry for love through all she did in her day. She caught a glimpse of it and her life is still full but she is different inside that life.

THE TO-DO LIST

I'm not saying for one second that there are not things to be done in the day! My goodness no! I live in the same world as you with a to-do list that is never all crossed off. And I LOVE to cross things off lists… just as an aside, I used to love crossing things off lists so much that if I did something in a day and it wasn't on the list, I'd add it to the list so I could immediately cross it off and look at my list and feel even happier that I'd gotten even more done in my day! The problem is not the tasks to complete. It can be the attitude with which you approach them that influences your health and behind that attitude is a belief. If you have eight hundred things on your to-do list, you can either approach it with an amped up, stressed out, freaking out on the inside attitude, or you can *feel* your feet connect to the earth, take a breath in and out that lasts for more than eleven seconds, and acknowledge that you have eight hundred things on your to-do list. Your headspace, whether it is pent up or calm, does not change what you need to get done in a day. It is what it is. But you can *choose* your approach. For calm and centred to become the natural centre of gravity from which you operate, you need to practice. You need to support yourself with lifestyle choices that promote calm (such as not relying on three double shot lattes to get you going in the morning) and explore what has led you to live in an anxious state. Is it physical/biochemical, such as too much caffeine before lunch, is it emotional, or is it both?

THE GOOD GIRL

When you curiously open the door on your racing around state, do you see that you are so scared of getting into trouble because you were raised to be a good girl ("goody two-shoes") that you live your life trying to do everything before anyone even asks you for it? Or before anyone yells at you for not having done it? Or so that no one will criticize you? There is no right or wrong here, no good or bad. This is not a judgment exercise on whether having a goody two-shoes aspect to your personality is a good thing or not. Our behaviours can serve us and also hurt us at the same time.

What I care deeply about is why you do what you do because then you can *choose* the behaviours that serve your health and the ones that don't can fall away. Until you explore the destructive behaviours in whatever areas of your life they appear, and get to the heart of them, change will be a battle, and you'll keep returning to your old patterns. Right now my concern is that if you live your life under the cloud of false belief that to never be rejected, you have to be little miss goody two-shoes—and while this will probably make you a kind and likeable person—it also runs the risk of making you a rushing woman, with all of the health consequences that go with that state when you live it long enough. The relentless pursuit of never being rejected… what is it costing you?

DADS AND DAUGHTERS

I'm going to make a big statement. From an emotional standpoint this is the biggest thing I'll say in the whole book. I have yet to meet a rushing woman whose father didn't break her heart. As an adult female, your father is either still your hero or he disappointed you (broke your heart) while you were growing up. You can of course as an adult bring awareness to this area of your life and find peace but my point is, with your father, it is was either one way or the other. Hero or heart-break. If he is still your hero, there won't be room for an intimate male partner to enter your life, or if you are in a relationship, he will play second fiddle to your dad; like whatever he does could never compare to what your father would do or what your father would have done. You will also not rush. You will still be your own boss. And you are in the minority of adult women. On the other hand, if your dad broke your heart, that disappointment might have appeared as big stuff such as death or abuse of any kind towards you or another member of your family or society. Or it may have been behaviours that hurt only you, that others may not have even noticed, comments that on the surface didn't seem hurtful but that could be *interpreted* that way. Perhaps it was an offhand comment that you cost a lot of money or one that hit a nerve with a client recently was "you're just like your mother." Maybe he was always late to pick you up. As a child you don't have the emotional maturity to understand that he may be late all the time because he is working hard to pay for the house you live in and the education he wants you to have so that you have the best opportunities in life. All you know is that he is never there when you want him. And that must be your fault.

A close friend of mine felt betrayed by her father and so angry with him for thirty-two years because he died from cancer when she was nine. As a forty-one-year-old woman she said to me "What kind of father leaves his nine-year-old daughter?" as if he'd simply walked out rather than passed away, making it sound like he had a choice. There she was in front of me as a grown woman speaking the words the nine-year-old felt. Because her dad died, her mum had to go to work, and my friend saw much less of her mum and financially their lives were more challenging after he passed. In my friend's eyes, through her lenses, she believed her dad abandoned her. And she also believed that money was scarce. One of the hardest workers I've ever met, and a woman with a relentless urgency about every aspect of her life, was created from that environment, which when you spell it all out on paper allows you to have great empathy for her. Of course she'd have those personality traits with that kind of past. As an outsider you can completely understand it and have immense compassion for her and how hard it must have been to lose her dad so young.

You too run behaviours based on your beliefs and I can guarantee you, if you've never looked at this before, you won't have any empathy for yourself. Instead, without realizing it, you will most likely judge yourself and treat yourself with impatience and harshness. Yet it is empathy and kindness towards yourself that you need in order to disarm yourself of the behaviours and beliefs that drive you to say yes to everything, to criticize yourself when you don't live up to the insanely high expectations you set for yourself, the guilt you feel at not calling your mother or your dearest friends enough, not to mention the emails you never reply to, and it is also why you've lost the ability to truly and utterly rest… all behaviours that hurt your health.

So when your dad, usually unknowingly, hurt your feelings and you created a belief that for him to love you, you had to be prettier, slimmer, taller, smarter, louder, quieter, more frugal with money, more generous, kinder, sweeter, worry less, care more… whatever you perceived his expectations to be, out of that, much of your behaviour has been borne.

Remember humans will do more to avoid pain than they will ever do to have pleasure. We are wired that way. We have to be to survive. And that is why when you live your life doing all you can so that your father, whether he is still of this mortal coil or not, will approve, be proud of you and therefore love you, you will be a rushing woman. Technology allows it. You choose it subconsciously, because a part of your nervous system was wired to do so, so that you will survive. Yet an adult, logical mind knows that living so stressfully hurts your health (as I've outlined in previous sections) and can lead to challenging relationships with the people you love the most in this world. So unravel your stories. And see them with new eyes. It is time to see the world as it really is, not through the eyes of your child self. It is time to take responsibility for yourself and your choices and understanding what drives those choices (avoiding rejection) changes everything.

As you begin to explore your stories (as opposed to reality), talk to yourself the way you would speak to a precious child, for with such tenderness, the fear of not being enough dissolves and is no longer the driving force of your behaviour in that moment. And the more consciously you live, the more you are present in each moment, you will so clearly see, that you are wonderful. There is not a little girl in the world who is not born knowing that she is wonderful. Not in a conceited way, just a precious kind of way. And we lose that. It is part of the human condition. Girls lose it at different times, but we all lose that knowing. And I believe we spend the rest of our lives trying to feel like that again, using food, shopping, achievement at work, or achievement at keeping people happy to do so. Yet if you knew who you truly are, you would be in awe of yourself.

The way Allison Pearson describes the "Dad thing" in her brilliant book *I Don't Know How She Does It* is with her main character Kate, a frantically busy wife, with a high pressure job in central London and two small children… and so much more, sharing this… "Now here's a funny thing. All the women

I know in the City are Daddy's Girls one way or another. Candy's dad walked out when she was five and I think she has been trying to find him ever since; Debra's ran a motor company in the West Midlands and was occasionally sighted by Deb and her sisters between rounds of golf at the weekend. Daughters striving to be the son their father never had, daughters excelling at school to win the attention of a man who was always looking the other way. Daughters pursuing the elusive ghost of paternal love. So why do all of us Daddy's Girls go and work in a place so hostile to women? Because the only real comfort we get is from male approval. How sad is that? How unbelievably sad is that?"

WHO IS AFFECTED BY RUSHING WOMAN'S SYNDROME?

When the enormity of the health consequences that arise from the perception of pressure and the need for urgency hit me, I first questioned where does it come from, what drives it, and who does it affect? I've outlined my take on these three questions above but as an addition to the third query I offer you this.

Initially when I reflected on the demographic affected by RWS I thought it was Western women in their thirties and forties but on observing patients with this in mind for the past five years, I can now very clearly see that most women are not immune to it. I've met women in their late sixties, some of the kindest, most caring, gracious women I have ever met in fact, who go into a panic on the inside as soon as anyone asks them to do anything. Two in particular spring to mind and they are both, individually, evidence that RWS is not just the result of the rapid increase in the technology available to us. Both of these women do not use email and both only bought cell phones to keep in touch with relatives overseas. They each saw me for different health reasons; one for weight loss and the other for such severe diarrhoea that when this lovely lady went for a walk in the mornings, she couldn't make it to the end of her street without having to run back home and use the toilet with an intense urgency. After tests with a gastroenterologist revealed nothing amiss with her bowels, I asked this lady about the relationships she shared with the people closest to her. She said her children were lovely (both were adults and lived overseas) but she merely tolerated her husband as he was a tyrant. He'd had multiple affairs that she knew about, and he raised his voice and overreacted at the slightest mishap. She appeared happy on the outside and yet on the inside she was wired and she did everything in her life with immense haste. She felt like she loved him, she said. The reality was she lived in fear of him, in this case not because of physical abuse but emotional. She said she chose to stay because she couldn't bear the thought of losing the home she had created over the past forty years. When I asked her if she felt like he loved her she said no and he hadn't for thirty-seven years and she'd done everything possible with her appearance, her body, her cooking, and her immense level of care in an attempt to earn his love. And the desire for his love spills over into the need to keep everyone happy… to keep the peace. And that's where the urgency, the rushing, and the intensity with which we as women approach our to-do list, comes from. Earning love. Never being rejected. Oh and too much caffeine. But I've barked on about that enough already.

I express no judgment here. I simply wanted to share a story with you to demonstrate that the rushing that has become part of the way so many women run their days is not just the result of technology and the immediacy that many of the devices we use today allow or "require" of us. Technology has simply made it easier for people like me (health professionals) to see it. If you try to fill something that can't be filled with what you are using, the emptiness never goes away and you keep wanting more. Only you usually don't see this until you explore your inner world.

Beliefs and thoughts lead to feelings and feelings lead to actions. Feelings can also lead to beliefs which then lead to actions. We respond to other people, treat our children, mates, strangers, coworkers and people on the street based on our beliefs. Everything we do, every word that we utter, every relationship we have is an expression of what we believe. A lady, Sonia, who works with me part-time recently told me she wished she could work with me full-time and forever. I giggled and asked her why and she replied because I am always happy, I talk to her kindly, and I laugh with her. I asked her what it is like at her other jobs and she said they hardly ever smile and mostly don't speak to her unless they have to give her instructions. And it made me wonder where courtesy and kindness are disappearing to in this world. And it led me to write this on Facebook...

There is a story behind every person. There is a reason why they are the way they are. Do your best to consider this always, as it helps us to not judge others.

The Dalai Lama says it beautifully when he says: "The basic foundation of humanity is compassion and love. This is why, if even a few individuals simply try to create mental peace and happiness within themselves and act responsibly and kind-heartedly towards others, they will have a positive influence in their community."

And Tony Robbins shared: "The more you recognize the best in others, the more gratitude you have for the gifts that make them precisely who they are. The more you express that gratitude, the more alive and fulfilled you feel—and the more you're able to appreciate the best in yourself."

NOT ENOUGH

The belief that you are not, and don't have, enough might manifest in unkind behaviour towards people you actually love. It may manifest as a desperate feeling for more... more of anything or anyone... which might show up in your life as eating too much, spending beyond your means or frequent, brief intimate encounters. A belief that you don't have enough will make you utterly blind to, and entirely callous about, those who have less because you believe that you are one of them. When you are caught in a trance of deficiency, your task, your only task, is to do whatever it takes to get more. If fortune throws a significant amount of money in your lap you won't see it. You will find a way to make it disappear so that the world you live in will be congruent with your beliefs. With decades of experiments examining everything from the efficacy of wrinkle creams to observations of car colours, scientists have discovered that we don't believe what we see, rather we see what we believe. Again, we don't believe what we see... we see what we believe.

Until you are willing to name your beliefs, either because circumstances force your hand or because you wake up to the pain of seeing through shattered lenses or because you are sick of living your life in a great big rush and the subsequent health consequences, you will continue to act on your self-created version of reality, which is why women who believe that all men cheat will see "evidence" of it in the way he interacts with every female he comes into contact with, even though he adores her. It is why lottery winners tend to blow through their cash and end up broke… even with millions they believe they are poor, and actions always conform to beliefs. Unless you name your beliefs you will continue to believe that your version of reality is the way that it is, not the way you choose it to be based on your beliefs. Naming beliefs and exploring the feelings that arise is an ongoing, exciting, heart-opening process.

AWAKEN THE PART OF YOU THAT IS ASLEEP

There are times when rushing serves a brilliant purpose and when it is short-lived, there is no problem for our physical and emotional health. We cope without a hitch. But when you live in that state day after day, year after year, it can take an immense toll on your health. And I've written this book because when I work with women and can see that the rush is at the heart of the health problems they've come to see me about, they firstly either deny they are stressed despite their blood tests showing they are and tell me this is just how their life is, or they agree to slow down ("funny you say that, my mother always tells me to slow down," they'll say) but they don't. Nothing about their lifestyle changes. And the best diet in the world, the best supplements, or the best exercise plan, won't even touch the sides when your sympathetic nervous system is always dominant. And to allow your parasympathetic nervous system, the rest and digest arm, to do it's vital work, you first need to understand what SNS dominance is actually doing to you and therefore *why* you need to change and then, secondly, you need to explore your emotional landscape of why you feel the need to do everything with urgency. As you now understand from the previous chapters in this book, we have very ancient hormonal mechanisms in action inside our bodies that believe they know better than you when it comes to your survival. Your body can be your biggest teacher if you learn how to decipher the messages it is communicating to you. And your behaviours, extra body fat or an unjustified panicked perception of life, are sometimes simply vehicles of communication, doing their best to remind you to rest the part of you that is weary and awaken the part of you that is asleep. And mostly the part of women that has gone to sleep is our belief, our deep knowing of how precious we are and that we deserve nothing but the best care, the utmost of kindness and nurturing, and nourishment for our body, mind, and soul; gifts we can choose to give ourselves every single day.

And for the mothers in particular, the women for whom guilt has become a way of life, I ask you to remember this sentiment... you are the best mother your child will ever have. You are their barometer and their compass in this world. And every single child thinks that their mother is absolutely wonderful.

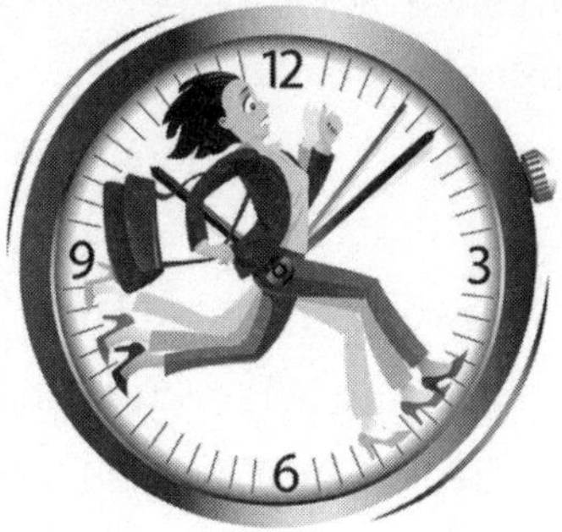

Chapter 6
What is it costing you?

It is with even more love and respect for women everywhere that I write this chapter. I believe many women are unaware of what living as a Rushing Woman is doing to them on a physical level—PMS, debilitating menopause, IBS, poor sleep, "unexplained" weight gain—as well as on an emotional level—feeling anxious, mood swings, anger, impatience, and easily laying blame for things on other people. And it is all of this that can easily lead a woman to dislike herself, judge herself, and hold a tension in her body that is destructive to her health and her relationships... not fun and lighthearted stuff which is partly why I opened this chapter with a gentle statement. Women are truly amazing. And they can do anything. My concern is that for so many women, their perceived need to be all things to all people is taking its toll in a much bigger way than most women may realize.

PMS

The link between stress and PMS is undeniable from both a scientific perspective and also my experience with clients. And as you now understand, when your adrenals are churning out stress hormones, your body does not feel like the world is a "safe" place and to keep you and the human race safe, so you won't bring a baby into your stressful world, the adrenal production of progesterone is compromised. Of course pregnancy can still occur when you are stressed as our emotional and primal drive to reproduce is also very powerful. However, with the amping up effects of adrenalin combined with the loss of the antianxiety agent progesterone, you have a biochemical recipe to rush and the basis of PMS.

As was outlined in the sex hormones section, the other biochemical picture that leads to PMS is estrogen being dominant to progesterone, not necessarily due to poor adrenal production of progesterone but through excess estrogen. Once estrogen has done its job in your body over a month, the liver decides whether to excrete the estrogen or recycle it. Recycling is far more likely when the liver has to prioritise the detoxification and excretion of substances that the body perceives as far more toxic to our health than estrogen. The body doesn't see estrogen as a poison because your own ovaries and fat cells make it. However, due to our environmental exposure to estrogens and estrogen-like substances, such as those in plastics and pesticides, not to mention synthetic versions of estrogen found in the oral contraceptive pill (OCP) and hormone replacement therapy (HRT), we are being exposed to more estrogen than ever before in human history. Combine that with women's increased intake of some of the major "liver loaders" which include alcohol, caffeine, and some refined sugars such as sucrose and high fructose corn syrup and any of its derivatives, and you have an additional recipe for the rush and another form of PMS due to a congested liver.

ANGER

The congested liver scenario presents an additional factor that can bring chaos into women's lives and their relationships... anger. I do not believe that any emotion is bad. The way we express different emotions can, however, be constructive or destructive; our expressions of emotions can either serve the world or not. Combine the feelings of impatience, frustration, and anger welling up inside a woman who perceives there are not enough hours in the day to do all she needs to do—which subconsciously she believes she has to do so that she will keep everyone happy and that her life depends on this—with a congested liver, a whole pile of stress hormones, often with negligible progesterone, and while we are at it, let's throw a couple of adrenalin-inducing coffees in and a dusty head from too much alcohol the night before, and you have a woman on the verge of becoming a cyclone at any conceivable moment. And when she lets fly, it will most likely be over something that in the big scheme of things doesn't really matter. Like the butter being left out or a wet towel being left on the bathroom floor. And who is most likely to be on the receiving end of her explosion? The people she loves the most in this world: her family, her flatmates, or her colleagues. Mostly, it is family. And as the beautiful Buddhist saying goes: "You will not be punished for your anger; you will be punished by your anger."

If the description above rings true for you, if you scream at your children or your beloved and wish you didn't, and if this is harder to control in the lead up to your period, please understand that the cocktail of hormones described above are powerful and likely to be behind your PMS-based anger. Secondly, if you drink wine, stop. Stop for three months. Your liver is screaming at you to change your ways. This is even more important if your breasts form lumps easily and if this is worse premenstrually. If taking a break from alcohol feels impossible to you, double check that this is the case. It is, after all, only a drink, and three months is a tiny amount of time in your long life. If you still say it is impossible for you, then switch to gin or vodka with soda, and add fresh lemon or lime. Measure the nip of spirits and limit it to two per day making sure you have a minimum of two AFDs per week. Also apply the strategies for estrogen dominance outlined in the solutions chapter. And thirdly, please understand that you need to make some changes, not only for yourself and your physical health, but also for the sake of those you love. They don't understand what is behind your outbursts. They think it is about them and that they have to change who they are for you to love them. Our children need us to take responsibility for our behaviours and, as you now understand, your behaviours are simply the outermost expression of your beliefs.

ALCOHOL

I meet women who truly believe that there is nothing harmful about drinking twelve bottles of wine a week. There is not a woman on the planet whose body, mind, or soul can handle that much alcohol, week after week. Most women I meet overdrink—that is they consume amounts of alcohol deemed by scientific research to be unsafe. Unsafe in relation to what? Most notably cancer. Scientific research has unquestionably linked the regular, overconsumption of alcohol to six of our major cancers: breast, colon, stomach, liver, throat, and esophageal. It worries me enormously the way so many women, both of child-bearing age and those who are postmenopausal, regularly overconsume alcohol. Please wake up and make a change in this area before a health crisis demands that you do. You don't need this book or a health professional to tell you that you drink too much if you do. You know better than anyone else. So now please let your own intuition drive you to make a behavioural change.

How do you do this? You pick an avenue to start. For example, you might choose to begin with the way you eat. When you eat an alkaline diet, your desire for alcohol decreases significantly. So you could commit to basing your diet on green plant food (and adding small portions of more concentrated foods; see the Alkalinity chapter in *Accidentally Overweight* for more detailed information) and watch your desire for both alcohol and sugar fall away. Or you could simply decide to take a break from drinking alcohol for one month. Or two. Or three. I've had women who initially felt like this would be impossible, do this without blinking an eye. And feel so proud of themselves for doing so. And then if you choose to bring alcohol back, drink only one or two days a week and not every week. Or save it for super special occasions. Or you can approach overdrinking from an emotional perspective. Ask yourself to finish the sentence "Alcohol is..." or "wine is..." and keep going until you get goose bumps (pimples), which signal that you have hit on your truth. And you will see that you have constructed a story about what this drink is to you. So then ask yourself what the other ways you could feel this way are. And bring more of that into your life. Or simply see that you subconsciously created a story about alcohol and why you "need" it, to get you through a tough time. It's just that you kept using it this way and now it is the only way you know how to, for example, relax. You have not always relied on alcohol to relax. There are plenty of other ways. Besides, when you rush less, which you will once you have gotten to the heart of your matter (emotions chapter) you will feel far less amped up and stressed and you will "need" alcohol to relax far less often. In fact, you will look at your life differently, through a different set of lenses, and see that a relaxed state of mind is available to you at every given moment.

The following is an article I wrote for a January edition of a women's magazine, just so you have some more facts.

Alcohol

As the festive season draws to a close, the effects of too much alcohol may still be silently, or loudly, reverberating. Whether it is increased body fat or cellulite, less energy and vitality, worse bouts of PMS or mood fluctuations... or perhaps your get up and go has got up and left, alcohol may be to blame. As fun as it can be at the time, alcohol can rob you of your clarity and purpose. And so January often sees us making big statements about our health and alcohol reduction or avoidance. Some wait until February to take a break, as they've worked out it has the least number of days! I know others who do Oct-sober in October.

We drink for wide and varied reasons. For some, it is the way they socialize, or the way they wind down from the day. Some use alcohol to distract themselves from thoughts and feelings they'd rather avoid. It can be a way that people cope. Regardless of the reason, many of us overdrink without even realizing it.

A standard drink is one hundred grams of alcohol in whatever form that comes. In New Zealand and Australia one hundred grams of alcohol is a 330-millilitre bottle of 4 percent beer, a thirty-millilitre nip of spirits, 170 millilitres of champagne, and it is a measly 100 millilitre of wine—about four swallows! Next time you pour yourself a glass of wine, measure it, and see what your natural pour is. For most, it is considerably more than 100 millilitres, and, as a result, many of us are overdrinking without even realizing.

The current recommendations provided by heart foundations say that for women, no more than two standard drinks per day with two alcohol-free days (AFDs) per week is okay, while for men, three standard drinks per day and two alcohol-free days is acceptable.

We have long heard the heart-health benefits of red wine publicly sung, and somehow it justifies to us that drinking is okay—you are clearly looking after your heart. Also consider the American Cancer Society's position statement on alcohol. It is very powerful and they "recommend" even less is consumed: two drinks maximum for men and one drink maximum for women per day, with a minimum of two AFDs per week.

I'm not suggesting you don't drink alcohol if that is your way. Alcohol consumption can be immensely pleasurable for those who partake. I simply want to appeal to you to get honest with yourself about how alcohol affects you. You know in your heart if you drink too much and when it is negatively impacting your health. Alcohol can also affect the way we relate to those we love the most in the world, and of course it affects how you feel about yourself. So, if you drink, consume your beverage of choice mindfully and certainly enjoy it, rather than for the misconstrued message that alcohol is good for your health.

The link between the consistent, over-consumption of alcohol and breast cancer is undeniable. Research has shown this time and time again, and for many years now. Yet we rarely hear about it. The American Cancer Society suggests that "even a few drinks per week may increase a person's risk (of breast cancer)."

The human body cannot excrete alcohol; it has to be converted into acetaldehyde by the liver, and then the acetaldehyde can be excreted. This is the nasty substance that can give us a headache the day after a big night. If the liver doesn't do its job properly and alcohol accumulates in our blood, we can go into a coma and die. Alcohol is that poisonous. And I don't say that lightly. But, thankfully, our liver jumps to action and starts the conversion process and we can carry on. Over time, though, this can take its toll.

The trouble is, when we drink daily, or, for some, just regularly, the liver can be so busy dealing with alcohol as its priority, that other substances that the liver has to change so they can be excreted don't get any attention and are recycled. Estrogen and cholesterol are two examples. It is often the reabsorption of these substances that leads to their elevated levels in our bodies—and that can lead to health challenges.

If you want to cut back or cut out alcohol for a while, or even if you just want to break your habit of regular drinking, still pour yourself a drink at the time you would normally have a glass of wine, and do what you would normally do. Sit and chat to your partner, make dinner, talk on the phone to a friend. So often we have mentally linked the glass of wine to a pleasurable activity when it is actually the pleasurable activity that we don't want to miss out on! So have sparkling water in a wine glass, with some fresh lime or lemon if that appeals, and add a few more alcohol-free days to your life.

~~~~~~~~~~~~~~~~~~~~~~

Please get honest with yourself about how alcohol affects you and those around you. And with kindness towards yourself, always kindness, take steps to drink way less than you do now, if this has rung true for you. From a calorie perspective, one glass of wine is the equivalent of three slices of bread. And I've met
~~~~~~~~~~~~~~~~~~~~~~

countless women who tell me that they couldn't possibly eat a slice of even good quality bread in their day, yet they will drink one-half to a full bottle of wine (or more) many nights of the week.

This is part of a vicious cycle. Because when you wake with a dusty head, many women will reach for coffee to clear the dust, another liver loader and adrenalin-production enhancer. Change these two dietary behaviours alone, and women will naturally rush a whole lot less and enjoy the health benefits that come with less urgency in their lives.

The following is an email written to me by a patient, who I will call Elise, who came to see me for help with her PMS. She said it was so bad that, even though she had a lovely husband, she wanted to divorce him for two weeks out of every month. She was prepared to do whatever I asked her, she told me, if it would help her be relieved of her PMS, yet when I asked her to take a break from alcohol for two menstrual cycles, she resisted. However, to her credit she did it and this is part of the email she wrote to me at the end of what turned out to be three very insightful months. I have Elise's permission to reproduce this part of her note.

> *"When you asked me to take a break from alcohol for two months I felt like crying. Instead I did what I always do, as you*

pointed out, which was to get angry. Three months have now passed and I cannot tell you how different I feel. I never really dreamt that I would be free of PMS. But it is gone. The thing is, part of me is devastated at what I used to be like. Thank goodness for my husband because he keeps reminding me that the way I used to behave can all be in the past now. But I'm horrified at what I used to be like. And I couldn't even see it. But now I see it in other women. Some of them are my friends. They scream at their kids at a level that is not OK. Children don't understand that there is a substance that changes your personality. They just know you are you and that you are their whole world and that sometimes you seem different and to a child that means that they must have done something wrong. I don't want women to think I'm judging them because it is as if they can't help it, let alone see it. But at the same time, though, I think they are behaving like a child themselves for not taking responsibility for their actions. If alcohol is what is behind someone yelling at or ignoring their children then they need to stop drinking."

The Dalai Lama offers brilliant insights about anger. He says it is a blind energy that (momentarily) destroys the part of your brain that is able to judge right or wrong. He says anger can't see reality. He says that to face a problem, we must know reality and the mind needs to be calm to investigate reality. Otherwise we can't see objectively. To use human intelligence properly, the mind needs to be calm. Anger destroys inner peace and the ability to investigate reality. And Elise's road to have the "blindness" reversed was dietary change, a significant part of which was not consuming alcohol for a period of time.

A raised voice, regardless of its intention, signals to a human nervous system that there is danger. If we yell at a child to warn them of danger, they get the message. If a child is yelled at because they dropped a glass by accident and then the next day they are on the receiving end of another raised voice because they forgot to take their drink bottle to school and then two days later they are again yelled at for not dressing themselves warmly enough, a pattern starts to emerge in their life, and they form beliefs about who they are, about what kind of person they must be to be on the receiving end of harshness from someone who is always right: their parent. Please, please, please know this is not designed to elicit guilt. It is designed to wake you up if this is part of you that has gone to sleep or is blinded by your anger. Please move beyond guilt if that is where you have gone in your head and hear my point. My point is that it is incredibly hard to express kindness when you feel broken. It is very difficult to practice patience when you are under immense time pressures. Yet patience and kindness are crucial here.

My cry to you is to please get your health, starting with the liver loaders, on track so that you can give your mind every opportunity to be calm. I believe that is our duty, that this is part of our responsibility to our children. And that is how you change the world.

Here's how to recognize that the liver needs support.

INDICATIONS YOUR LIVER NEEDS SUPPORT

- Liver roll—that increased roll of fat high up under the bra of women, under the pectorals of men.
- Tender point in the centre of your torso (can indicate gall bladder issues, heartbreak, or massive disappointment); if your gall bladder has been removed, your liver has to make the bile the gall bladder once did, so additional liver support is often required.
- Very short fuse or temper

- Episodes or feelings of intense anger
- "Liverish," gritty, impatient behaviour
- PMS
- Cellulite (lymphatic or cortisol related also)
- Overheating easily
- "Floaters" in your vision
- Waking around 2:00am
- Sleep which is worse on an evening you consume alcohol
- Waking hot in the night
- Not hungry for breakfast when you first get up in the morning
- Prefer to start your day with coffee
- Elevated cholesterol
- Estrogen-dominance symptoms
- Bloat easily
- Drinking alcohol daily
- Daily long-term caffeine consumption

IBS

Irritable bowel syndrome or any other digestive system disorder can make being intimate with the person you love, the least appealing thing on the planet. And without going into enormous details here, most husbands link physical intimacy to you loving them. And sure they might understand for a couple of days that you aren't in the mood, but when those few days stretch into him perceiving that you haven't felt like being physically intimate with him for years, that can be tough on a relationship. Not to mention that you can also miss out on the closeness and pleasure. So if your tummy problems are the way your stress and your SNS dominance play out, explore whether this is having an impact on your wider life. What does it mean for you socially? At work? Are you always on edge making sure there is a toilet nearby? Do you decline special invitations so you don't have to risk having an upset tummy and so miss seeing people who uplift you? I know many women who have searched for years to solve their battle with a bloated or unpredictable tummy. So please know ladies, there is a reason. And as I outlined earlier, the most common ones are SNS dominance, a parasite infection/gut dysbiosis, or a "food intolerance". Or two or three of these factors. So apply the suggested strategies and have your tummy no longer be a source of your discomfort and interior panic.

DEBILITATING MENOPAUSE

If a woman has been in SNS dominance for many years and then her sex hormone production starts to change, her menopause is far more likely to be challenging and potentially debilitating, with some of the major symptoms being hot flushes, interrupted sleep, and vaginal dryness. In this section, given the focus on what being a rushing woman is costing you, I simply want to encourage you to see that it is crucial to sort out the RWS drivers before going into menopause so you are more likely to experience more subtle changes in your health parameters and the way you feel. Going into menopause with SNS dominance sets you up to have poor adrenal production of progesterone, the hormone with significant antianxiety and antidepressant properties. Once menopause arrives, ovarian production of hormones ceases and in an ideal world, you would go from having good progesterone production to a small amount from your adrenals glands. Instead, what I see every day of my working life, are women who go from having a progesterone reading of "<0.5" (so virtually zero progesterone on a day of their cycle when ideally there would be 25 units of progesterone) to the same super low reading in menopause. Without good adrenal production of progesterone you have nothing to fall back on when ovarian production ceases. So sort out the rush before menopause begins.

If you are currently passing through menopause

and you went into it with all of the classic signs of RWS, there is still so much you can do to support your health. These strategies are outlined in the solutions chapter. And if you are now postmenopausal and still feel panicky on the inside, again the strategies outlined in the next chapter will serve you. There is so much you can do to support your health. I encourage all of my clients to see their body as a barometer. Your body does not have a voice but it will always give you symptoms to let you know if it is unhappy and wants you to pay attention to something. And often it is to your very own intuition.

POOR SLEEP

What is living in SNS dominance costing you? Often the quality of your sleep. And when our sleep quality is compromised, so many aspects of our health are impacted upon. When you are unrefreshed from your sleep, you tend to make poorer food choices; most often you will reach for the high-sugar foods and/or caffeinated drinks believing you need them to keep going. So poor sleep can affect your desire to take good care of yourself.

When we don't sleep well, long-term, all of our pituitary hormones can also be affected, which as you now know can affect every cell of your body. Thyroid hormones, sex hormones, and of course stress hormones have been found to be higher in those who don't sleep well. The flipside of that is also that adrenalin, one of your stress hormones, does not want you to sleep as it is communicating to every cell of your body that your life is in danger so the last thing it believes is that it is safe for you to sleep deeply. When I see patients who have come to see me for help with their sleep, the majority of women are SNS dominant and until we can alter that, the deep restful, restorative sleep that people once knew does not return on a regular basis. You need to do all you can to allow your body to feel "safe." And sleep will come.

Poor sleep also has a relationship with your other stress hormone, cortisol. As was outlined in the stress hormones section, cortisol levels naturally fall away in the evening and allow you to fall asleep. Cortisol naturally starts to rise around 2:00am, and sleep is less likely to be as deep after this time. Going to bed by 10:30pm, at the latest, is ideal for restorative sleep. But what rushing woman is going to do that?

EMAILS

I'll say it again... when you tell me that you delete emails off your phone while sitting on the toilet because that's good time management, I can tell you, with love and respect, that you are a rushing woman. Emails can infiltrate every corner of your life if you allow them.

I was recently able to witness New Zealand women's Internet habits when I announced that I was holding a second cooking school (the first one sold out in two hours prior to this one being announced). The announcement went out via email at around 4:50pm and with a limited number of seats, I had to watch the sales carefully. The initial influx of sales happened up until around 6:00pm. My guess was that women then either drove home from work or began preparing dinner. There were very few sales between 7:00pm and 8:30pm and then, within the next hour, the event was all sold out. And it made me think... where once, after dinner, women connected with the people they love, did household tasks, read or relaxed, they now finish their evening duties and head to their computer to do emails, use social media, or do more work that they brought home from the office. Where once, weekends were for recreation, connection, shopping, gardening, and perhaps solitude and time for reflection, now the work, the emails, and the social media use continue. Or if it doesn't continue, it is often on a woman's mind so that by the time she gets to Sunday, if she hasn't done any of these things over the weekend, women will tell me that a mild panic sets in with the anticipation of what will be in their in-box the next day. No nervous system on the planet can handle panic long-term. Sure there are times when emails and social media are great fun and bring us pleasure. But when they compromise your health because you dread the sheer number of emails or what they will contain, there is a bigger thing at play, and the emotions section of this book is crucial for you. Too much time spent on your computer can cost you precious moments with the people you love the most in this world. It's just that we forget to notice this along the way.

BODY FAT

A Rushing Woman may be slim, skinny, or overweight. In *Accidentally Overweight* the focus was on the nine factors that determine whether humans use body fat as their fuel effectively or not. So to capture a part of the essence of that message that is particularly relevant to RWS, I offer you this:

It is as if many women's bodies never feel "safe" enough to use fat as fuel for they are constantly on red alert, ready to act the split second the next "crisis" happens. Humans burn fat effectively when we have what I call a balanced nervous system and, as you now know, that is when we can switch appropriately between being SNS dominant and PNS dominant and also sit comfortably and happily in what is known as homeostasis… when your body is in balance. Create the "safety," re-establish optimal health, and the body fat burning will naturally and effortlessly follow.

If you are now even more busting to know how to reestablish a balanced nervous system, many strategies are offered in the final chapter.

TO SUM UP THIS CHAPTER…

This was the hardest chapter to write because some of what I felt needed to be expressed will be hard for some of you to read. I intend no offence, no judgment, no guilty responses, only insights and experiences from my work and my amazing clients. I want you to be happy and I want you to experience amazing health. I want you to truly know, feel, and experience the incredible woman that you are. It is time to treat yourself with the care you deserve.

The following is a gorgeous piece written by the talented Kate Northrup, a woman with a deep care for other women and who I met at a conference in the U.S. recently. She wrote this on a piece of paper and found it in her car when she cleaned it not so long ago. Her sentiments echo many of my own. I encourage you to be inspired by her words and to create your own "Here's what I know…"

HERE'S WHAT I KNOW...

- Doing something for the money never ends up being worth it
- If it's not a hell yes, it's a no
- You are valuable because you exist. Period. (Or, full stop if you're British)
- You are enough. You always have been. You always will be
- Your place of greatest ease and joy will also be your place of greatest service
- It's okay to sleep for ten hours or more a night from time to time. In fact, it's critical
- No accomplishment or moment of recognition will ever replace feeling loved, by yourself or anyone else
- You know. You always know
- The fact that it feels good is reason enough to move every day. The fact that it will tone your ass and make your waist smaller are mere side effects
- Organizing your life around what feels good is the single wisest choice you can make
- Saying yes to someone simply because you don't want to disappoint them is not only unfair to you, it's unfair to them

- Sleep, water, movement, greens, and a good cry cure almost anything
- Anything worth taking seriously is worth making fun of. (Thanks, Mom)
- Paying attention to your money is a profound act of self-love
- It turns out that life is happening right now
- Loving yourself more is the best place to start to solve any problem
- You can't judge and have an open heart at the same time
- Nothing is random. Everything happens for a reason
- Your body is wise beyond what you could possibly imagine. Listen to her. She will lead you home every time
- Home is not a place

Your turn!

What do you know?

What can you count on no matter what?

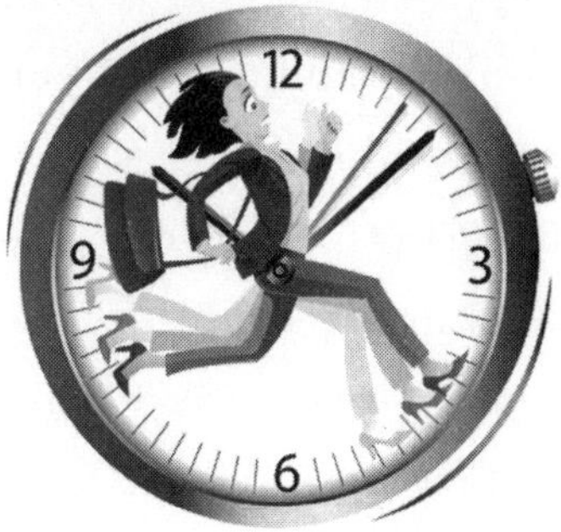

Chapter 7
Solutions

It is always tempting when reading a book to jump straight to the solutions, especially for a Rushing Woman! When you think that you don't have the time to read the whole book, you just want to cut to the chase and get the answers, then put answers into action and get your results. Right? Umm, well hear me out.

If you've come to this chapter first, I cannot encourage you enough to return to the beginning of this book and read it from cover to cover. Science teaches us, and I am certainly convinced from working with people for fourteen years, that you first have to know *why* you need to change something for when the why is strong enough, the change is a natural follow through. If the solutions offered here were simply a list of instructions, then this section will only be additions to your never-ending to-do list that you may (or not) do for two weeks or two months, but before long you will return to your old ways and the health consequences that potentially go with them. Without knowing why I might be asking you to focus on your breathing every day for the next six weeks, you might do this for a brief period but as soon as you get beyond busy, you will feel like you don't have time and the breathing sessions will cease and the rush will begin again... if it ever stopped in the first place. So to that end, you need to know *why* I am making the following suggestions.

Secondly, there are suggestions scattered through each chapter that won't necessarily be repeated here. Thirdly, I believe that you are more likely to take action to care for yourself when a particular section of this book speaks directly to you. When that happens, when you feel like I've read your diary or your mind, or like I've caught a glimpse of your life, or perhaps you got goose bumps, laughed, or cried, then you are far more compelled to act, than if you simply read my recommendations below.

I begin with a set of suggestions designed to help your biochemistry switch from rushing to calm. And I remind you to please spend some time in solitude, with a journal by your side if that appeals, exploring what may have bubbled to the surface for you while reading the emotions chapter, in particular. Once you catch a glimpse of where the rush originated, the immense power to change your whole life is in your hands, and change naturally flows from this space.

Small changes can have powerful results. Imagine that your life's destiny was going to run like a set of railway tracks, with the left track remaining a consistent width apart from the right track. Let's say these imaginary tracks are set to run from New York to Dallas. From the point you begin to make lifestyle changes, even if you only change what you do or how you think by two degrees, the left and right tracks will start to veer away from each other. At first they are just a few metres (feet) apart but after a few months they are kilomitres (miles) apart and after a year, you are worlds apart from where you would have been had you not initiated change. The right track, the path of your previous destiny, will still arrive in Dallas. However, by adopting your changes and sustaining them, the left track will now arrive in Miami. Worlds apart.

Restorative Eating

It is very difficult to be kind, compassionate, and patient with others when you fill yourself with stimulants and foods that contain very little nutritional value. I believe that if each individual embraces compassion, kindness, and patience, there will be no need for violence in any form. But if humans fill themselves with too much caffeine, alcohol, and "dead" food, it makes it much harder for them biochemically to consistently access these gentle emotional states. A real food diet allows you to explore your emotional landscape with clarity and free yourself from patterns that no longer serve you.

Food becomes part of you and the nutrients from food drive every chemical reaction inside of you. Choose real food that nourishes you and watch your physical, as well as your emotional, health shine.

- Eat real food
    - Nature gets it right
    - Human intervention does not
- Unprocess your diet… Zigzag if you need to
    - Eat food the way it comes in nature as often as you can

    - Relax on Fridays and Saturdays (for example) if you want to
    - When you are in control of your food, you "zig" and eat nourishing food; when you are at someone else's house for dinner (for example) you eat what they serve and you "zag"... that way you still get to socialize without compromising your health
- Double the amount of green plant foods you currently eat
    - Add a green smoothie for breakfast or for a snack
    - Take nutrient-dense leftovers for lunch instead of buying a sandwich that will likely only have a token amount of greens on it
    - Stay tuned for the release of my upcoming support system of recipes designed to help you amp up your greens called *The Real Food Chef*
- Cut out or significantly limit caffeine
    - Take a break from coffee, black tea and caffeinated softdrinks (soda) for four weeks

    - After that, if you want to bring it back only drink it when you go out for breakfast or perhaps on the weekends… remember it is what you do every day that impacts your health the most, not what you do sometimes… your rituals create your life
    - This is crucial for a rushing woman as her adrenalin levels are usually already high enough
    - Still go to your favourite café but instead choose green tea or herbal tea or a dandelion tea (made like a latte), or less often a decaf (make sure it is Swiss water filtered to limit your consumption of the usual chemicals used to decaffeinate coffee beans—most cafes have the Swiss water filtered decaf these days), or order a green juice
- Cut out or significantly limit alcohol
    - Get honest with yourself about how alcohol affects you and those around you

    - If you drink it every day, it stops being special
    - Drink only on special occasions
    - If you drink every day it is too much
    - If you consume more than 200mL of wine a day and have less than two AFDs per week, scientific research suggests you are damaging your health
    - Swap alcohol for sparkling water with fresh lemon or lime
    - If you want to keep drinking, swap wine for gin or vodka and soda with fresh lemon or lime for four weeks; less alcohol (you tend to have one standard drink instead of three per glass), less sugar, no preservatives... all liver loaders
- Follow the digestive system strategies outlined later in this chapter to maximize nourishment

Restorative Movement

If you are SNS dominant from the way you live your life, adding more factors to your world that promote SNS dominance will not solve your rush.

Remember, you often resist the most, what you need the most. I witness this in my work with people every week of my life. If you are currently into loads of cardio, you may tell me that yoga will "bore you to tears." I call cardio "yang" exercise and I describe some forms of yoga as "yin." Most rushing women need to incorporate more yin movement into their lifestyle on a regular basis. I also encourage women to do some form of regular resistance training whether that be using weights or simply using their own body weight.

Yin movement includes:

- Qi gong
    - A delicious way to start the day
- Restorative yoga
    - If there is one form of movement that is truly nourishing and replenishing for rushing women, it is this. It truly lives up to its name. The poses are simple to learn and easy to incorporate into your daily life (see more detail later in this chapter)
    - It is particularly beneficial for those who identified with the pituitary depletion, the adrenal depletion, or the thyroid depletion health pictures

    - It is also outstanding at regulating the menstrual cycle and for fertility
    - It is the most divine, feminine, restorative movement I have discovered
- Meditation
    - The stillness that comes from regular meditation is in itself a journey and a reward.
    - If your mind is super busy find a CD you like that can guide you. It can help to have someone talking or asking you to imagine things for a period of time when the meditation first starts. And then once the mind is quieter, you will embody the stillness on offer
    - Meditation takes practice
    - We understand that we need to train the body; you can't run a marathon without any training. You have to work up to the distance with practice runs. The mind is the same. It takes practice to train it
    - The following is a piece written by a

lady who had resisted meditation but stuck with it:

"Today I had my usual pang of anxiety about the future and getting sick, being in an accident, losing someone who is close to me (my mind is incessant; it never stops), but then something amazing happened. I just let myself fall into the feelings and the whole thing opened up. I had read about this before but never experienced it. I felt like the entire night sky, filled with stars, was inside me. It was really amazing being able to witness a moment of terror and pain transform into something calming and expansive."

- Feel your feelings; part of growing up is learning that your feelings will not destroy you. They are just feelings. And they too shall pass

- Daily gratitudes
    - When you are grateful you cannot be stressed
    - Say out loud or write down each day at least three things for which you are grateful. I gave you many examples

throughout this book if you don't know where to start

  - It can be gorgeous to keep a journal to capture your gratitudes and any other murmurings that bubble to the surface while you are in this space. Insight often comes this way and we get clarity about something that perhaps we felt confused about

- Some form of yin movement needs to be incorporated a minimum of three times into your week. Ideally set up a daily ritual. But if that means starting out with a once a week session then that is wonderful. Yin begets yin!
- If you insist on continuing to cardio it up every day, start your day with a yin ritual such as qi gong

Restorative Sleep:

As discussed earlier, there are a few things I link to amazing health. Optimal nutrition, of course, fresh air, movement, love, forgiveness, and great sleep. Sleep affects our physical and mental health enormously. Sleep is often the only time our PNS can dominate, and I suspect that for many women who don't sleep well, it isn't even happening overnight. It is vital that you schedule maximum sleep time for yourself if you want to start feeling bliss from the inside out. Restorative sleep is critical to every level of our health. Of course, if you have little ones that need you during the night, support yourself to sleep when you can, and remember to breathe and remind yourself that they are little for such a short time.

If you do not sleep well or you do not feel restored after sleep, apply any (or all!) of the strategies below. The overall concept here is to do whatever it takes to get you to stop churning out adrenalin.

- Omit all sources of caffeine for eight weeks
    - That includes soft drinks and chocolate as well as the obvious sources of tea and coffee
    - Wean off caffeine if you currently have more than two caffeinated drinks per day, by having a green tea daily for three days and then omiting
    - After eight weeks, if it has helped, you choose whether you bring it back or not
- Omit alcohol
    - You may feel like it helps you fall asleep but it tends to disturb most

people's sleep patterns during the night as it prevents you from going into the restorative, deep REM sleep

- Do not sit in bright light for two hours before you want to go to bed
- Get up at the same time each morning and expose your eyes to sunlight. Light destroys your sleep hormone melatonin and allows your happy, calm, content hormone called serotonin to surge
- Avoid doing work for a minimum of two hours before bed and engaging your brain in this way
- Consider the age of your bed
    - Dust, mould, and sweat all accumulate in mattresses plus beds lose their support. You spend one-third of your life in bed so it is best to make it a place that brings out an "ahhh" moment of bliss when you fall into it each night. This "ahhh" moment alone is good for your health!
    - If your bed is more than ten years old, it is most likely not supporting you well and the waste accumulation

may be affecting your health. This is particularly true if you experience allergies to dust, mould, and/or asthma.

- Schedule (and do!) twenty long slow deep breaths daily
- Do restorative yoga poses daily
- Meditate and/or pray regularly

Restorative actions:

Feeling like your life has purpose and meaning is crucial to restorative actions. Contribution is key here. When you make a difference in someone else's life, your heart feels fulfilled. As the poet Rabindranath Tagore so beautifully said: "I slept and dreamt that life was joy. I awoke and saw that life was service. I acted and behold, service was joy."

- Pick up any litter you see
- Call people you may not have caught up with for ages—they will be thrilled
- Volunteer
    - A male friend of mine who works in more than a full-time job was standing on a street corner collecting money for the City Mission. Among many things, they raise money for food to feed

people on Christmas Day. My friend said he does a half day for them every month and I had no idea. He'd never mentioned it. He said it was the least he could do because he has so much

- Bake a cake and deliver it to an aged care facility and stay a while and talk to the residents; you will make their day and you will learn something
- Give the clothes you no longer wear to an organization who can use them
- Smile while you walk along the street
- Notice the colour of the sky wherever you are
- Send someone a card in the mail to let them know you are thinking of them
    - My amazing mum has sent me an envelope packed with bits and pieces every week of my life since I left home to wherever I am in the world! It is usually filled with pictures from magazines she has collected that she thinks I will like and the births, deaths, and marriages from the local paper from my hometown. It always makes my day. Thanks Mum.

- If you think of something that amuses you and you think it would entertain someone else, tell them, text them, and share the giggles
- If you see someone looking lost ask them if you can help
- Practice random acts of kindness
- Be kind. As I love to say, kindness must come first

We are all connected

I once met a rushing woman who was beyond stressed. And when I asked her why she told me it was because she had twenty-three Christmas presents to buy before Christmas and it was already November 24. I thought she must have had an overwhelming number of other commitments between now and Christmas but she said she didn't. No work, nothing major scheduled, no major family dramas. Without judgment, I gently suggested to my client that she needed a reality check and asked if she had ever considered how blessed she was to firstly have twenty-three people to buy for and secondly to have the financial means to pay for these gifts. I watched her face respond like a typical rushing woman with expressions of guilt and realized that sometimes we get so caught up with ourselves that we forget we are part of a greater whole.

Something very special unfolds in our lives when we remember that we are part of a universe that connects all things. For when we recall that, it often fosters a desire to contribute to the world beyond our own immediate gain. I find the happiest and healthiest people are often those making a difference to what I have come to call "the greater good" in ways that are meaningful to them. When we turn up to a job each day that we don't really like and that is jam-packed with pressure, yet our perception is that to be responsible we must stay there, I find that engaging in activities that are meaningful to you somehow eases the pain, pressure, and exhaustion of that work, especially if the work is not meaningful to you. I've also met countless people who have quit financially rewarding jobs to spend a year or the rest of the foreseeable future doing something that is more meaningful to them. Do something you care about. Sometimes sadness crops up in an attempt to wake you up to your passion. I am not suggesting for one second that you quit your job. I'm simply suggesting you find a way to contribute to the world around you and witness a part of you wake-up to the joy that has always been there.

Radiant Living

There are many different forms of yoga and yoga means different things to different people. I find people gravitate to yoga for a wide variety of reasons. For some it is movement. For others it is a spiritual practice. For some it is a path to stillness. Some begin because they developed a degenerative disease such as cancer. For others it is just a cool thing to do; all of their friends are doing it. For others it is a preventative health practice and for others it is part of their spiritual journey. For many it is how they bring balance into their very hectic lives. In yoga circles they talk of the Sages 10 Rituals of Radiant Living. I encourage you to embrace them in ways that are meaningful to you.

1. Ritual of Solitude
2. Ritual of Physicality
3. Ritual of Nourishment
4. Ritual of Abundant Knowledge
5. Ritual of Personal Reflection
6. Ritual of Early Awakening
7. Ritual of Music
8. Ritual of Spoken Word
9. Ritual of Congruent Character
10. Ritual of Simplicity

Keep a Journal

Buy yourself a beautiful notebook that can be your journal. Capture anything you like in there. Be sure to express your gratitude as a daily ritual. If you feel like you don't have time, keep it in the living room or the kitchen… some place in your house where you will see it. Keep a pen with it or, better still, some coloured markers and whenever you clap eyes on it, think of something for which you are grateful and write it down!

Stop, Keep, Start

Another great thing to do with a journal is to make a list with the following headings:

- Stop
- Keep
- Start

And fill each column in as you think of things by answering the questions:

- What am I going to stop doing?
- What am I going to keep doing?
- What am I going to start doing?

You can use the suggestions on these pages to give you ideas. Here is a sample:

Stop: I am going to stop getting caught up in gossip as it is exhausting

Keep: I am going to keep eating a nourishing breakfast every day

Start: I am going to start walking four days out of seven for the next two weeks starting tomorrow morning at 6:00am

Stop, keep, and start goals can make change fun, manageable, and suitable for your lifestyle.

Exploring Your Inner World and Emotional Landscape

The peace you seek is within you. To help you explore your inner world, to begin inquiry, to help you understand your subconscious reactions more, to help you lose the emotional charge from a relationship that in your head you are over, but yet your body still seems to react... Try any of the following:

- NSA
    - This stands for Network Spinal Analysis but the name does not do it justice
    - NSA involves gentle precise touch to the spine which cues the brain to create new wellness promoting strategies. Two unique healing waves develop with this work. They are associated with spontaneous release of spinal and life tensions, and the use of

existing tension as fuel for spinal re-organization and enhanced wellness

- Practitioners combine their clinical assessments of spinal refinements with patient's self-assessments of wellness and life changes

- Greater self-awareness and conscious awakening of the relationships between the body, mind, emotion, and expression of the human spirit are realized through this popular healing work. NSA is exclusively practiced by chiropractors

- The Journey
    - Created by the gifted Brandon Bays, this process (described in her book of the same name) allows you to "see" the world as it really is, rather than the stories you have constructed around things. It allows you to see the beliefs that no longer serve you and allow them to effortlessly fall away. And as you now understand when your beliefs change, your behaviour changes as your behaviours are the outermost expression of your beliefs

    - The Journey is a powerful healing tool through simply fostering the innate healing within you

    - It would not surprise me if one day science can show what many people already believe to be true and that is that cellular changes can be fostered through thought. I truly believe this to be the case

- The work of Tony Robbins
    - Tony's book "Awaken the Giant Within" is brilliant. Don't just read it… do the exercises in it!

    - Tony's live event Date With Destiny is powerful beyond measure. He is a genius. His work (also available on CDs) allows you to see and then change your limiting beliefs and the emotions you so desperately want to avoid and foster those you want to experience. His work, his contribution to the world, has forever changed the face of psychology and helps people, no matter how massive or relatively small their past hurts may have been, move forward into an empowered future

- Restorative Yoga
    - I personally had never experienced such deep stillness before restorative yoga became part of my life. The gracious, kind, and insightful Tracy Whitton was my first teacher of this beautiful practice, and I am eternally grateful to her for developing what she has come to call "*Stillness Through Movement.*" Thank you for sharing this with the world, beautiful lady
    - It consists of yoga poses, pranayama (extension and control of the breath), breath awareness exercises, and meditation (training the mind in openness and kindness). The technique helps restore the body/mind connection
    - Stillness through movement is a process where one learns to align with one's true consciousness/intelligence (rather than the stories)
    - Through breath and mind awareness

one is able to let go deeply allowing you to receive the benefits of the restorative pose, bringing the body/ mind back to its natural state of peace and contentment

- Without this awareness you tend to live in a permanent state of unease, so when you practice in this way you begin to align with the ease of life. Your new saying might just become “Life is simple and easy!”
- The parasympathetic nervous system is effectively activated during restorative yoga. As you now know, the PNS is responsible for balancing the body and bringing its response system back into equilibrium. Restorative yoga takes the spine and nervous system out of the “flight, fight or freeze” response, relaxing and calming the adrenals
- To do this props are used to support the body so no strain occurs, yet you can hold any posture anywhere from two minutes to twenty minutes. It is sometimes referred to as “active relaxation”

- Some poses target a certain area or gland, such as the pituitary, where others have an overall benefit. All poses create specific physiological responses which are beneficial to health and can reduce the effects of stress related disease. In general restorative practice is great for those times when one feels weak, fatigued, or stressed from day-to-day activities or for those who find other styles of yoga too difficult

- These poses are especially beneficial for those times before, during, and after major life transitions like: death of a loved one, change of job, pregnancy, marriage, new baby, children leaving home, divorce, or adrenal burnout. You can also practice the poses when ill or recovering from an illness or injury. Or simply incorporate them into your life on a daily or weekly basis

- It is great for re-balancing hormones in women who have PMS, challenging puberty, menstruation, or menopause

- What is also exceptional about restorative yoga is it doesn't matter whether you have never experienced yoga before or have been practicing for thirty years. This yoga can guide you to where you need to go. I personally LOVE it

The Serenity Prayer

Don't worry about something until it's a problem. If it becomes a problem, then you can face it, but worrying about something that truly may never happen only serves to hurt you. As we now know, stress, whether it is real or perceived, may promote the production of excess cortisol and drive SNS dominance. The ripple effect of a worry can very slowly and subtly change your mood and your metabolism. And it's the chemical signals of your body that are driving this. The beautiful, old piece of wisdom called "The Serenity Prayer" is useful to remember and act on, especially if you are a worrier:

God, grant me the serenity to accept the things I cannot change,
Courage to change the things I can,
And the wisdom to know the difference.

And as Geneen Roth so eloquently says: "Every time

you stop fighting with the way things are, you return to yourself, to heaven on earth. Can you stop fighting today? Can you give yourself that much of heaven?"

There is great freedom and a slice of heaven in acceptance.

USEFUL TESTS TO EXPLORE YOUR BIOCHEMISTRY

To examine your "rushing" biochemistry, to explore your hormones levels thoroughly, you can visit a health professional and have your blood and/or saliva tested. Useful blood tests include:

- Thyroid group:
    - TSH
    - T3
    - Reverse T3
    - T4
    - Antithyroid peroxidase antibodies (anti-TPO)
    - Antithyroglobulin (anti-TG)
- Adrenal:
    - Cortisol: urinary twenty-four-hour collection or first morning collection

- Ovarian (some are also related to pituitary function):
    - Estrogen
    - Progesterone
    - LH
    - FSH
- Vitamin D: many people are deficient in this crucial nutrient. Have yours tested and supplement if it is low. It is involved in countless, vital processes in your body
- Cholesterol (is the building block of your steroid hormones and elevated levels indicate that the liver needs support—see liver support strategies below)

If your results come back out of the "normal" range or skewed one way, strategies are offered below for each of the groups above (for cholesterol employ the liver support strategies). It can be very useful to seek guidance from a health professional to guide you specifically. Just because your blood tests come back "normal"if you exhibit all of the symptoms for dysfunction with a particular gland, find someone who will work with you to treat your symptoms rather than your blood work. I have clients all over the world who fall into this category.

The body gives us symptoms to communicate to us that it wants us to live differently; perhaps eat differently or think differently. I believe in every moment we are given a second chance.

STRATEGIES TO ASSIST YOU SECTION BY SECTION...

FOR THE NERVOUS SYSTEM

The Nervous System has been presented as its own chapter. This was important to help you see the way your nervous system controls and influences such a wide variety of aspects of your health. If I simply asked you to slow down you'd tell me I don't understand how demanding your life is. So I needed to explain sympathetic nervous system dominance in detail. The whole goal of this book as well as the following strategies is to assist you to spend far more time in your daily life with your parasympathetic nervous system being dominant or certainly to allow the two arms of your nervous system to be balanced and respond appropriately, rather than the SNS always running the show, for in this latter scenario, our health on every level is compromised.

More Generalised Solutions...

- The way you breathe is key, even though that sounds too simple to make a difference

- Start the day with twenty long slow breaths before you get out of bed or, alternatively, breathe and move your diaphragm while you wait for the kettle to boil, or while you sit at traffic lights
- Enrol in a breath-focussed movement class two to four times a week, such as tai chi, qi gong, or restorative yoga
- Start the day with movement, followed by an egg-based breakfast for two weeks, and notice if this sets your day up better
- Swap coffee for green tea (except if you have problems with sleep… see earlier suggestions) and notice if you feel calmer and more energised an hour later after a week of doing this
- Add more fat to your meals, particularly lunch, in the form of avocado, nuts, organic butter, tahini, oily fish, and observe if your desire for sweet food mid-afternoon diminishes. That way you can choose a healthy afternoon tea, rather than be ruled by that "eat your arm off feeling"
- If you recognise that you do tend to try

to be all things to all people or perhaps you walk on egg shells around a boss or a family member who at times has an explosive temper... consider seeking the assistance of a health professional with this and learn how to change the way you approach these situations. The patterns mostly get set up in childhood. My suggestions include:

- Seeing a Journey practitioner
- Consulting with an NSA (network spinal analysis) practitioner
- Go to Date With Destiny or read *Awaken the Giant Within*
- My Essential Women's Health Weekend and/or DVD
- Seeing a cognitive-behavioural therapist-trained (CBT) psychologist
- Seeing an NLP (neurolinguistic programming) practitioner
- Seeing an EFT (emotional freedom technique) practitioner

FOR THE ADRENALS

How high your level of stress is and how you feel

your body copes with it will influence the steps you take. The above section of solutions is general, and I can confidently say that virtually everyone will benefit from applying them.

The herbs used for adrenal support are beautiful, however it is best to check with a qualified medical herbalist to find out about herbs that will meet your specific needs. I have made comments beside most of the herbs about their applications.

If you have identified that you are adrenally fatigued and beyond exhausted on a daily basis, your adrenal support is listed separately, and restorative yoga would be extra wonderful for you.

Solutions For Adrenal Support

- Schedule and commit to regular breathing exercises. It can literally change your life. And I do not say that lightly

- Practice yoga, pilates, tai chi, or qi gong a minimum of twice a week for four weeks. Develop a daily practice for outstanding results

- Spend five minutes daily focusing on and giving voice to all the aspects of your life for which you are grateful; you can't be stressed when you feel grateful

- With the guidance of an herbalist, take some

adrenal support herbs. I am not associated with any brands of supplements, but when I have good reason to favour one I will mention it. When it comes to herbs, nothing compares to Mediherb, an Australian-based company (products available internationally) with the highest of standards. I mostly use liquid tinctures and, at times, the tablet combinations. The majority of these adrenal herbs are adaptogens, meaning they help the body adapt to stress by fine tuning the stress response. They include:

  - Withania, for the worriers
  - Rhodiola, for the drama queens or occasionally for the worriers
  - Siberian Ginseng, for the fatigued feminine
  - Panex Ginseng, for the utterly fatigued
  - Licorice, especially if your blood pressure is on the low end of normal
  - Dandelion leaves, especially if you retain fluid

- The adrenals also love vitamin B and vitamin C, and for adrenal support I usually supplement both: the Bs in the form of a multivitamin (I highly rate USANA's Multi-Essentials; proven scientifically to have the best absorption of any multi available, plus it has great results clinically for people) or a straight B complex, plus 4-5 grams per day of vitamin C, preferably in powered form with added calcium and magnesium. If you are on an oral contraceptive pill, stick to 2 grams of vitamin C per day

- Just as important, if not the *most* important aspect of supporting adrenal function for a balanced and appropriate stress hormone response, is the application of the emotional health strategies (explored in the emotions chapter) and breathing

Adrenal Fatigue Supplementation

As I outlined in the magazine article included in the adrenal chapter (included the information here again so you can find it easily), for people with deep, deep fatigue, I almost always use the following herbal tonic that contains:

- Panex ginseng
- Licorice
- Dandelion leaves

- Astragalus
- One other herb depending on what else is going on for the individual (a liver herb or a reproductive herb are typical)

I will also sometimes use a range of supplements from the United States created by Dr. James Wilson specifically for adrenal fatigue. I have had countless clients take this range of supplements for three months and have their energy and vitality return to great levels.

The Restorative Power of Real Food

Although I often recommend good quality supplements of herbs and/or nutrients for adrenal fatigue (and other health conditions), never underestimate the healing and restorative power of food the way it comes in nature. Taking supplements is not a reason to eat a poor quality, low-nutrient diet. I simply recommend high quality supplements where appropriate and especially to assist in the restoration of health.

For Peri- and Postmenopause

As I said earlier in the book, if you are peri- or postmenopausal, I can't encourage you enough to address adrenal health and liver health for these two systems, as well as the overall balance of your nervous system, tend to make all the difference to your menopause symptoms.

FOR SEX HORMONE BALANCE

Menstrual Cycle Challenges

- If you have any type of menstrual cycle or reproductive system challenges, take a four-week break from alcohol or, better still, take a break from it for two menstrual cycles. You'll see your PMS significantly decrease
- If this solution is "impossible," decrease alcohol intake to two nights a week, and preferably drink less than half a bottle of wine
- Coffee can be another big-ticket item when it comes to PMS, via liver congestion. Consider swapping coffee for green tea for four weeks, or preferably two menstrual cycles, and see how you feel
- Take a four-week strict break from all dairy products

For estrogen dominance (which can be confirmed with a saliva or a blood test):

- Extracts of broccoli or broccoli sprouts. I am all for getting what we need from our food, but, in this case, you need to eat eight heads of broccoli a day to get the same therapeutic effect as one good quality capsule of broccoli extract

- For PMS, the following table is useful. You may experience one or a number of different PMS patterns at once

Menopause strategies

- For hot flashes consider whether the heat is coming from low estrogen, liver/gall bladder congestion, or both?
  - For low estrogen, Black Cohosh and Sage can be useful.
  - For the liver/gall bladder, Globe Artichoke, St Mary's thistle, Bupleurum, and Schisandra are excellent
- For adrenal support, Rhodiola can be brilliant if you are also exhausted or Siberian ginseng or Withania
- For low blood pressure, Licorice is excellent
- Magnesium

For all the challenges discussed in this chapter, focus on the gifts of your feminine essence.

The different types of PMS:

the mechanisms involved, and the potential treatments

	Symptoms	Mechanism	Potential Treatment
PMS-1	Anxiety Nervous tension Irritability Mood swings Insomnia	Elevated estrogen Low progesterone High cortisol	Vitex Dong quai Vitamin B DIM
PMS-2	Water and sodium retention Abdominal bloating Weight gain Breast tenderness	Elevated aldosterone (fluid) Low dopamine	Dandelion leaves Vitamin B Vitex Rhodiola
PMS-3	Craving for sweets Increased appetite Can't resist refined sugar, followed by palpitation and fatigue Dizziness, shakiness, headache	Low magnesium Deficiency of prostaglandin PGE1 (low in an anti-inflammatory substance) Elevated insulin	Magnesium Essential fats; UDO's oil or fish oil or a flax oil and evening primrose oil combination Cinnamon
PMS-4	Period pain and clots	Elevated prostaglandin PGE2 (pro-inflammatory; increases inflammation in the body) Deficiency of anti-inflammatory substances Possible magnesium deficiency	Bupleurum if clots Dong quai Magnesium Essential fats, fish oil, flax oil if vegetarian

FOR YOUR THYROID

- Go on a grain-free diet trial for a minimum of four weeks
- If you *love* dairy products and the idea of going without cheese makes you wonder if you could, then do it! Remember, it is often what we love (not just like) to eat that can be a problem. Do a four-week dairy free trial if this is the case
- Support liver and gallbladder function to assist with bowel elimination. Globe artichoke is particularly good for "thyroid" people
- Refer to the advice about estrogen dominance
- Adrenal support is almost essential, especially when beginning to treat the thyroid. Refer to the stress hormones chapter to refresh on adrenal support strategies
- You will probably crave coffee. Please explore taking a four-week break and observe how you feel at the end of this period. Use green tea, which has a low caffeine level, instead
- If you have a diagnosed, underactive thyroid condition and you are on synthetic medication but your symptoms are still

present, explore transitioning to whole thyroid extract under medical supervision

- See a health professional to be guided about what minerals will be best suited to meet your individual needs. For example, you may need additional iodine, selenium, iron and/or essential fats
- Explore how you can change the "demands" on your time if you have an overactive thyroid by revising the thyroid and emotions chapters

FOR YOUR PITUITARY

- Restorative yoga
- Herbs:
  - Vitex
  - Alfalfa
  - Ginseng family
  - Licorice
- Oils: sandalwood, clary sage, massaged into soles of feet and/or reproductive organ areas

When the pituitary is at the heart of someone's problems (please understand I am not referring to pituitary diseases) they will often have suboptimal health with a number of endocrine organs which may include the ovaries (sex hormones), the adrenals (stress hormones), and/or the thyroid (thyroid hormones). When I suspect the pituitary needs some support I will tend to use Vitex in a woman who is menstruating and Rhodiola post-menopausally for "pituitary people." People with a pituitary that is not functioning optimally from too much SNS dominance will often feel better addressing adrenal, ovarian, and thyroid function. Pick one and start there. Or simply start with the pituitary by doing restorative yoga.

FOR YOUR DIGESTION

Digestion is central and essential to every process in our body. It is the base on which we build. So, whether your aim is to slow down, weigh less, optimize your health and well-being, and/or improve a challenging or diseased gut, or all of the above, understanding your digestive system is a crucial step to optimal health.

Remember to:

- Slow down! Chew your food
- Include fats and/or protein with each meal as you are likely to eat less and be satisfied with less total food for that meal, than if you simply eat carbohydrates on their own

- Eat less. Reduce your portion size by one quarter, especially in the evening if you overeat, and see how you feel
- Wake your stomach acid up before you eat by using lemon juice in warm water or apple cider vinegar before meals, breakfast in particular
- Drink water between meals, not with meals
- If efficient bowel evacuation is a particular challenge for you, reference *Accidentally Overweight* and the numerous strategies outlined there
- Omit a food you feel you cannot live without for a trial period of four weeks. The first four to seven days will be the most difficult but persevere. The results may be enormously worth it
- Working with a wonderful practitioner of Traditional Chinese Medicine can also assist you in healing your gut
- Try Aloe Vera juice to start your day if you have a particularly irritated gut
- Eat in a calm state
- Look at the food while you eat it. Do not read or watch TV while you eat

- If you suspect a parasite infection, the herbs Black walnut and Chinese wormwood are excellent as is oregano oil
- If you suspect you have some not-so-nice gut bacteria that are fermenting your food, apply all of these strategies first to see if that helps as often the bad guys have been able to take over because of the pH of the large intestine and this is mostly influenced by what goes on higher up the in the digestive system. If these strategies don't work, trial a probiotic supplement that is only Bifidobacterium species
- If you suspect you are reacting to a food, omit that food from your diet for a period of four weeks strictly. If it makes no difference, bring it back. If it helps, leave it out for three months and then try it again. Or if you are happy to go without it, then do so. If it is a food that is a rich source of nutrients, for example, gluten-containing foods tend to be a good source of B vitamins, then you will need to supplement. It will also be necessary to supplement with a mineral supplement that contains a combination of calcium, magnesium, manganese, boron,

and vitamin D if you omit dairy products. This is of lesser importance if your diet is plant-based and highly alkaline. It is best to seek the guidance of a health professional with this last point and particularly if you are going to omit food/s to get a resolution of your symptoms

- Chamomile is one of the best remedies for constipation and complete evacuation. This because it softens the waste and helps the bowel wall relax. Either drink lots of tea, or take capsules with each meal

Another remedy is one that many people have strong opinions about—colon hydrotherapy or colonics as they are known. This process involves a tube being inserted into a person's rectum through which warm or cool water gently flows. It allows the hardened faecal matter to soften; just like heavy, consistent rain works on dried out soil, allowing the large bowel to empty fully, getting rid of built-up waste that may have been there for a very long time. I have had clients tell me that the waste they excreted during their first colonic was black, implying that it may have been there for many years, interfering with healthy bowel function. One lady told me she saw popcorn in the "viewing" pipe during her colonic and she knew that the last time she ate popcorn was the last time she was at the movies... six months ago!

Colonics polarize people. The idea either appeals to you or it doesn't. There is no middle ground with people's love or dislike of colon hydrotherapy. I will encourage you, though, to not lose sight of what trends have done to medicine. Up until the early 1900s, colon hydrotherapy was part of general medicine, and doctors understood the importance of good bowel evacuation. In fact, coffee enemas were actually cited in the Merck Manual for Doctors for liver detoxification until 1972. It is a very personal choice. When you examine the history of medicine and observe the split between what we now know to be Western medicine and complementary medicine, it is clear why this happened, however this book does not seek to explore this segregation in detail. I will simply say that colonics were once accepted as a very "normal" treatment method for a host of health conditions, not just bowel issues. With a well-functioning bowel, an enormous load is not only taken off the digestive system but also the liver, the organ primarily responsible for cleaning our body. Help prevent bowel cancer by ensuring efficient bowel evacuation using methods that suit you! Always seek advice from a health professional before undertaking colon hydrotherapy if it appeals to you.

FOR YOUR LIVER

If you identify that your **liver** health needs to be addressed to assist you stop rushing and reacting with anger here are some solutions for your liver:

- Set yourself a time-based goal when it comes to making these changes. For example, "I will only drink alcohol on weekends for four weeks," or "I will only drink coffee when I go out for breakfast on Sundays."
    - Take a break from alcohol
    - Only drink on weekends; no alcohol during the week
    - Replace coffee with green or white tea (or, less often, weak, black tea)
- Support the liver with herbs such as:
    - St Mary's Thistle, especially if alcohol is a regular part of your life
    - Globe artichoke, especially of you have a tendency to constipation and/or a liver roll (fat roll under your bra) and/or central torso tenderness
    - Bupleurum, especially if there are clots in the menstrual blood
    - Schisandra, especially for its detox action (it also works on the adrenals)

- Transform anger into passion by giving a different meaning to a past experience; the energy of anger and passion are the same
- Drink vegetable juice or a "green smoothie" each morning
- Snack on seeds and nuts
- Eat less fruit; none after morning tea
- Cut out dairy products for a four-week trial and/or
- Cut out grains (containing gluten) for a four-week trial
- Take an essential fatty acid supplement; a good quality, decent dose of fish oil for reducing cholesterol, or a flax oil, evening primrose combination
- Eat high zinc foods such as oysters (from clean waters) or take a zinc supplement of zinc picolinate 15 to 30 mg per day and best taken at night just before bed to maximize absorption

Remember, it is what you do every day that impacts your health, not what you do sometimes. Just get honest with yourself. And take such good care of yourself that your quality of life is forever excellent. We only have one liver!

The Wrap-Up

My favourite quote spoken by His Holiness the Dalai Lama is this:

> *"When asked 'What thing about humanity surprises you the most?', the Dalai Lama answered: 'Man… because he sacrifices his health in order to make money. Then he sacrifices money to recuperate his health. And then he is so anxious about the future that he does not enjoy the present; the result being that he does not live in the present or the future; he lives as if he is never going to die, and then dies having never really lived.' "*

And it breaks my heart that this is true for so many people. I want you to live in love and from love and not in fear. It is crucial "you" don't disappear. The world needs you. And for you to be happy, for you to feel the joy, for you to be able to appreciate the many, many magical moments on offer to you, you so desperately need to slow down.

So, as I said I would, I've given you things to do to begin this process. And as Yoda says: "Do or do not, there is no try." I've given you strategies to bring calm and spaciousness back into your life. And I've had you thoroughly exploring, with kindness and curiosity, rather than judgment, what has led you to sacrifice your own needs and potentially your own optimal health and pursue whatever it was you thought you wanted... which remember is almost always the means to gain the love and approval of someone significant to you. And once you have caught even a glimpse of that... of what has been driving you, your life will never be the same again. You may still get caught in the rush sometimes, but you won't get stuck there and you certainly won't sacrifice your health. You'll find you have more of a voice if you have been more of a "keep the peace" kind of female because there has been a shift in your level of care for yourself and how far you will go to preserve that. Plus by always doing things for others, they never get to experience what it is like to give to you, nor do they get the opportunity to grow, if you always do it all for them.

But if you do get caught in the rush, you'll notice much sooner and you'll giggle and I hope you find it fun to explore what led you there that time. There is so much joy and beauty when you follow anything to its end.

I wish I could tell you that if the idea of applying strategies to combat your rush and the health consequences of your rush is not for you, then you could simply "do" the most feminine of "solutions"... and that is to simply be... I wish I could tell you that worked. But right now if you are juggling a million things and there are still a million unattended to, "being" ain't going to just happen. If all of the above feel overwhelming to you and like just another to-do list that you will never ever have all ticked off, then simply begin with two things: your long, slow diaphragmatic breaths and taking a break from caffeine. Commit to these daily for four weeks. Begin there.

And while you are at it, become so aware of what you say to yourself. Become aware of when you say cruel things to yourself and catch yourself. Work out what led you there. It will almost always be a feeling that led you to believe that you are not (good) enough and therefore won't be loved. And when you can see that is all it was and that now you are an adult, that you are "safe" and that the whole thing is nothing but an old outdated story you tell yourself, a little piece of you that has been asleep will wake up. And let that piece of you be the part that takes such good care of you for the world needs you... needs you happy and healthy to share your gifts with it! May you have a healthy body, an open heart, and a peaceful mind.

References and Resources

Here is a list of further information that may assist you on your journey. There are books and articles I've cited in the text, listed here if further reading in a particular area interests you.

Nutrition information is always changing and I am passionate about keeping you up to date with the latest and most insightful aspects of health and well-being. Please be sure to visit my website and register for this free service so you don't miss a thing! This service will also allow you to be informed about my live seminars, as I travel extensively and bring my message to life. It is my favorite thing to do.

After reading *Rushing Woman's Syndrome*, you may ask, what's next? I have had so many emails from people all over the world saying they feel like I've read their diary when it comes to describing how they feel in the pages of this book. People tell me they want more of this type of information and a specific program to follow that encompasses guidance with food, hormone balancing, and strategies that give them further insight into their emotional eating patterns. I cannot encourage you enough to check out the array of options on my websites.

My mission is to educate and inspire people and help them change the relationship they have with their bodies and their health and put the power of choice back in their hands.

So visit: www.drlibby.com

and

www.rushingwomanssyndrome.com

and continue your optimal health journey. I also post health information each weekday on Facebook and Twitter. Connect with me there at:

www.facebook.com/DrLibbyLive

www.twitter.com/DrLibbyLive

It is an honor to assist you.

Not all of the areas presented in this book have additional resources listed as I have read and studied widely (sometimes from very geeky biochemistry textbooks), and this book is the culmination of my knowledge, experience, observation, and intuition in this area to date.

Bennett, Jane and Pope, Alexandra. *The Pill: Are You Sure It's For You?* Sydney: Allen & Unwin, 2008.

Coates, Dr Karen and Perry, Vincent. *Embracing the Warrior: An Essential Guide for Women* Burleigh Heads, Arteriol Press, 2007.

DeVrye, Catherine. http://www.greatmotivation.com

Epstein, Donny. *The 12 Stages of Healing*. Amber-Allen Publishers. 1994.

Fasano, Dr Alessio *et al.* (2000) "Zonulin, a newly discovered modulator of intestinal permeability, and its expression in celiac disease," *The Lancet* 355 (9214): 1518-1519.

Hay, Louise. *You Can Heal Your Life*. Carlsbad: Hay House Inc, 2004.

Northrup, Dr Christiane. *Women's Bodies Women's Wisdom*. London: Judy Piatkus Ltd, 1998.

Northrup, Kate. http://katemoller.com

Pearson, Allison. *I Don't Know How She Does It*. New York: Anchor, 2011.

Robbins, Anthony. *Awaken the Giant Within. London:* Simon & Schuster Ltd, 1992.

Roth, Geneen. *Lost and Found: Unexpected Revelations About Food and Money*. New York: Viking Penguin, 2011.

Weaver, Dr Libby. *Accidentally Overweight*. Auckland: Little Green Frog Publishing, 2010.

Whitton, Tracy. *Stillness Through Movement*. Gold Coast: Tracy Whitton, 2011.

Whitton, Tracy. *One With Life CD*. Gold Coast: Tracy Whitton, 2011.

Acknowledgements

To my precious husband Chris Weaver... oh my goodness, thank you doesn't go close to expressing my gratitude to you and for you. Thank you for your authenticity, your eyes, your arms, for cracking me up, for your magnificent and very generous heart, and for teaching me so much. Thank you for your care for me, for the man that you are, and for helping me share my messages with the world. I adore you.

To the very lovely Kate Wilkie... thank you for sharing the busiest year of my life to date with me and for working along side me with such patience and grace. Thank you for your humour, your insights and observations, and for your care. You are such a special human and I feel very blessed to know you. And thank you for being the antithesis of a rushing woman!

To my dear parents... thank you for your unconditional love, and for your interest and support of my work. Thank you for the way you raised me and for being such wonderful people.

To my dear friends... Karen, thank you for your immense kindness, your raw and authentic emotion and for sharing you with me. To Leisel, thank you for the delight I feel in your company, the stories, and the laughter. To Petrea, thank you for your honesty, your care, your gift with prose and for being such fun. To Alexandra, thank you for our authentic conversations, your insights and your feedback about rushing women! To Karl, whose love of fabulous words inspires me to find more "good and nice" descriptives.

To Tracy Whitton, Neale Svenson, Craig Reynolds, and Jamila Cranston-Buckley for being exceptional at what you do, for having such an impact on my health and for having amazing hearts that you share with the world. Special mention and thanks to Megan Bardsley for her grace.

To Cynthia, the Real Food Chef... thank you for your enormous skill and passion for real food and working alongside me to create food, rushing women so desperately need!

To JoJo Brown for her beauty and humour... you embody the feminine and the tools you offer women to help them embrace their essence are powerful.

To Sharon and her delicious team at Gwinganna Lifestyle Retreat in Queensland, Australia... thank you for your friendship, generosity and for allowing me to "retreat" and begin the creation of this book in the nurturing arms of Gwinganna.

To my editor Caroline Webster… thank you for understanding my intentions with my writing, for your input and your appreciation of this manuscript. I value your contribution immensely.

Thank you to the very lovely Collette Moss, my amazing assistant who makes it all come together. I'd be lost without you.

Thanks to the very clever Garry Kewish for his unwavering support and guidance with my work. I am very grateful to you, Garry.

Thank you to Tony and Sage Robbins for their gifts of insight into the tremendous heart of real human psychology. I couldn't do what I do without all I've leant from all that you've shared. Tony you are a genius and I'm very grateful to you.

When I first caught a glimpse of what I have come to call Rushing Woman's Syndrome, I wanted to help women, the world over, calm down and take better care of themselves. I also want to take my hat off to them for all that they contribute to this world. You do all you do because of your deep care for people and this world. I simply want to help you to not do it at your own expense. Thank you amazing women of this world.

About Dr Libby

Born and educated in Australia, Dr Libby Weaver (PhD) studied at the University of Newcastle from 1993 until 2006. She completed a Bachelor of Health Science (Nutritional and Dietetics) with Honors in 1998 and went on to complete a PhD in the biochemical and nutritional factors affecting children with autism. Through this work Libby came to better understand, become passionate about, and communicate the relationships between the food we eat, our thoughts and beliefs, and the way our body then expands or shrinks.

Since 1999, Dr Libby has been working with individual patients from all walks of life, from stay-at-home mums to Hollywood stars. She set up and ran an organic café and she has been an integral person in the creation of two of Australia's major health retreats where she not only designed the nutritional philosophies, but also performed the role of Program Manager.

Dr Libby moved to New Zealand in 2007 to be with her husband Chris, since which time they have created a Holistic Nutrition Consultancy that provides people all over the world with consultations as well as empowering, informative seminars and retreats. Dr Libby is a regular columnist for many magazines including *Next, Good Health and NZ Life & Leisure*, and she is a passionate and sought after international keynote speaker. Her first book *Accidentally Overweight* became a best-seller within three weeks of being released.

www.drlibby.com

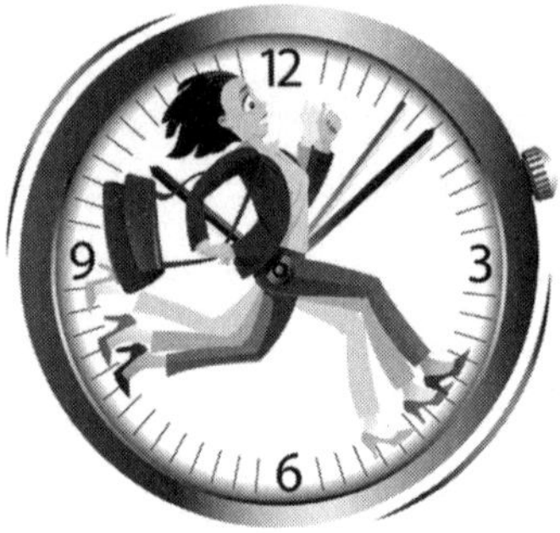